COPING SUCCESSFULLY W
IRRITABLE BLADD

JENNIFER HUNT is a lecturer in clinical psychology at
t_ _ _ _ _. O/P. retain 3/5/05
the NHS at W _ _ _ _
in health psychology, which she teaches to postgraduate
students. She has published a number of articles on bladder
problems and is researching in this area.

Overcoming Common Problems Series

For a full list of titles please contact
Sheldon Press, Marylebone Road, London NW1 4DU

The Assertiveness Workbook
A plan for busy women
JOANNA GUTMANN

Birth Over Thirty
SHEILA KITZINGER

Body Language
How to read others' thoughts by their
gestures
ALLAN PEASE

Body Language in Relationships
DAVID COHEN

Calm Down
How to cope with frustration and anger
DR PAUL HAUCK

Changing Course
How to take charge of your career
SUE DYSON AND STEPHEN HOARE

Comfort for Depression
JANET HORWOOD

Coping Successfully with Agoraphobia
DR KENNETH HAMBLY

Coping Successfully with Migraine
SUE DYSON

Coping Successfully with Pain
NEVILLE SHONE

Coping Successfully with Panic Attacks
SHIRLEY TRICKETT

Coping Successfully with Prostate Problems
ROSY REYNOLDS

Coping Successfully with Your Hyperactive Child
DR PAUL CARSON

Coping Successfully with Your Irritable Bowel
ROSEMARY NICOL

Coping Successfully with Your Second Child
FIONA MARSHALL

Coping with Anxiety and Depression
SHIRLEY TRICKETT

Coping with Blushing
DR ROBERT EDELMANN

Coping with Cot Death
SARAH MURPHY

Coping with Depression and Elation
DR PATRICK McKEON

Coping with Strokes
DR TOM SMITH

Coping with Suicide
DR DONALD SCOTT

Coping with Thrush
CAROLINE CLAYTON

Curing Arthritis – The Drug-Free Way
MARGARET HILLS

Curing Arthritis
More ways to a drug-free life
MARGARET HILLS

Curing Arthritis Diet Book
MARGARET HILLS

Curing Coughs, Colds and Flu – The Drug Free Way
MARGARET HILLS

Curing Illness – The Drug-Free Way
MARGARET HILLS

Depression
DR PAUL HAUCK

Divorce and Separation
Every woman's guide to a new life
ANGELA WILLANS

Don't Blame Me!
How to stop blaming yourself and other people
TONY GOUGH

Everything You Need to Know about Shingles
DR ROBERT YOUNGSON

Family First Aid and Emergency Handbook
DR ANDREW STANWAY

Overcoming Common Problems Series

Overcoming Common Problems Series

Overcoming Common Problems

COPING SUCCESSFULLY WITH YOUR IRRITABLE BLADDER

Jennifer Hunt

sheldon **PRESS**

First published in Great Britain in 1995 by
Sheldon Press, SPCK, Marylebone Road, London NW1 4DU

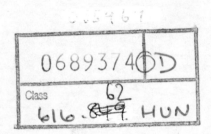

British Library Cataloguing-in-Publication Data
A catalogue record for this book is available from the British Library

ISBN 0–85969–717–7

Photoset by Deltatype Ltd, Ellesmere Port, Cheshire
Printed in Great Britain by Biddles Ltd, Guildford and King's Lynn

This book is dedicated to my parents,
with love.

Contents

Acknowledgements

I wish to thank the staff of the department of urological gynaecology at St Mary's Hospital, Manchester, for their help, particularly Sister Jill Lord, Dr Tony Smith and Gordon Hosker. Also all my colleagues at the department of clinical psychology at Withington Hospital, Manchester, for their encouragement, and a special thank-you to Dr David Unwin for his advice and support.

Introduction

You may be wondering if this book is for you. You have perhaps flicked through and seen a couple of diagrams and looked at the contents page. You are not too sure if you actually *have* an 'irritable bladder' and, even if you have, whether reading about it will help. So, I will start by explaining who this book has been written for and then will go on to describe how it could help you.

If your life tends to be planned around your bladder and, to a greater or lesser extent, it influences your daily life, relationships and activities and how you feel, then read on. Do you feel uneasy if you don't know where the nearest toilet is? Do you try to avoid situations where a toilet may not be within easy reach, such as travelling or going to the cinema? Are you constantly aware of how full your bladder is, how much you've drunk and when you last went to the toilet? If the answer to any of the questions is 'yes' then this book was written for you.

Irritable bladder, as I will use it, is a term that can refer to a variety of bladder problems. These can range from having to empty the bladder frequently when feeling nervous (something everyone experiences to a certain extent) to bladder pain and discomfort and even incontinence. Just like irritable bowel syndrome, which you may have heard of, there are several symptoms that you may experience. What irritable bowel and irritable bladder syndrome have in common is that medical treatments (drug therapy and surgery) are not always completely successful in relieving the symptoms. You may have had experience of this yourself. This book contains information about various simple approaches that can help as well as explaining common medical treatments.

Bladder and bowel problems have other things in common. The first, and most important, is that we find it enormously difficult to talk about them openly, even to doctors, and will try to keep them hidden from family, friends and colleagues for fear that people will judge us harshly and because we ourselves feel that the difficulties in some way reflect on our character or self-control. There is an unspoken 'taboo' surrounding bladder problems. This makes it difficult to discuss them and understand them. This is something that is

1

emphasized to us at a very early age and can make our experiences of such problems all the more upsetting and difficult to cope with. The second common factor stems from such difficulties in accepting and discussing these problems openly, which is that we do not realize how very common these symptoms are and what simple measures we can adopt to help us overcome them. This books aims to be educational, in the sense that how these problems can arise will be described and you will also be encouraged to design your own individual plan to improve and cope successfully with your symptoms.

So, how common *are* the symptoms we're talking about? Research has shown that at least 20 per cent of women have problems with frequency and urgency of urination. That is to say that one in every five women have difficulties, often feeling the need to pass water and having to visit the toilet a lot. I am constantly struck by the number of people who have bladder problems. When I have spoken to colleagues and friends about my interest in this area, they reveal personal experiences, such as having to get out of bed at night for 'one last visit', even if they have only been about 20 minutes earlier. Some of the people I have seen in the course of my daily work may have been passing water 20 or more times a day. Naturally, this is incredibly disruptive to everyday life.

If anything, the number of people with bladder problems is underestimated because, as we have seen, there is often a reluctance to reveal them. Therefore, any of the figures you see quoted are probably too low. Men and women of all ages can experience bladder problems, although men seem to have fewer difficulties, particularly with incontinence. For this reason, I am aiming this book mostly at women, although much of what I say will apply equally to men and I do give some specific information where it is relevant.

Estimates for incontinence vary depending on who is studied and how the questions are asked, but you may again be surprised to learn that over 30 per cent of adult women (that's one in every three) are occasionally troubled by incontinence and over 10 per cent are regularly incontinent. I hope you can see that if you are experiencing bladder problems you are certainly not alone. In fact, it is practically impossible *not* to know someone with similar problems, even if you've never discussed it with them.

It is difficult to say exactly how common incontinence is because defining the problem is not easy. Generally, it is defined as being an 'involuntary loss of urine'. As you can imagine, there is a great deal of variation in the amount and frequency of such loss. Also, the term itself obviously has negative associations and so people are often understandably reluctant to use it. Some may prefer to say they are damp or leak a little. I shall use the term 'incontinence' to refer to the unwanted loss of urine for clarity's sake and hope that any embarrassment you feel will be soon overcome. I will use words such as 'urinate' and 'pass water' to describe the act of emptying the bladder voluntarily. Other terminology will be described as we go along. Please do not assume this book is not for you if you don't suffer from incontinence. The book is aimed at coping with urgency and frequency, which can be part of incontinence problems but are also commonly experienced without it.

Why, then, is this book necessary? And why, you might be wondering, has it been written by a psychologist? First, let me explain my background. I am a clinical psychologist working for the NHS with adults who have health problems. I have a particular interest in bladder difficulties and am researching in this area. In my experience of working with patients with a wide variety of health difficulties, from diabetes and arthritis to headaches and heart disease, it is the person's reaction to their difficulties that determines how they cope, both practically and emotionally, which, in turn, can affect the course of the illness. There are no clear-cut distinctions between what is 'medical' or 'physical' and what is 'emotional' or 'psychological', even with very 'bodily' problems. Perhaps I should illustrate my point.

Two people, John and Julian, injure their backs in a similar way after slipping on some ice. Both are in a good deal of pain. Their doctors reassure them that nothing is broken or permanently damaged and prescribe some painkillers.

John is distressed, he has important deadlines to keep at work and cannot afford to have any time off because he is hoping for promotion. He was already feeling stressed and this is almost the last straw. He takes one or two more painkillers than he should and struggles to work. He manages in this way for two days and then is told to go home because people can see he is in pain and he is not working well. He is really down about his inability to struggle on and takes to his bed. The pain seems almost unbearable and he continues taking his painkillers. After two days in bed, worrying about work, the pain is still bad. He calls the doctor out. The doctor

3

is surprised that John is so distressed and wonders if he has missed something. He refers John for a specialist orthopaedic opinion and prescribes some stronger painkillers, thinking it will reassure him. John worries even more about his pain, thinking this could be something serious, and is really concerned about work. He tries to get up, but worries about aggravating the problem, so eventually stays in bed. He feels that things are out of his control.

Julian is also worried. He, too, has important things to do at work. He thinks about the pros and cons of struggling on and decides, for his own sake in the long term, it is important to take it easy for a week. He phones in sick. He stays in bed for a few days, reading and watching TV to take his mind off the pain. After this, he starts slowly to do more things, resting if the pain worsens. He is reassured that things are getting slightly better over time. He returns to work after a week and is careful not to overdo it. He feels in control and things are soon nearly back to normal.

These stories may seem a little exaggerated, but, I hope, you get the idea. A person's reactions (that is their thoughts and feelings) influence how they cope and recover. There are many factors involved in how a person reacts to bladder problems. If you can look at how you view things, then you are more able to change how you cope with them. Coping, or having a sense of practical and emotional control, can make an enormous difference to your daily life and can actually reduce the symptoms and distress you suffer.

People with long-term bladder problems naturally feel that their bladders rule their lives. You may find that you have adapted over time by avoiding certain situations or activities, but that the problem is often on your mind. Taking a step back to look at the problem can help you to cope with it more successfully.

Let me give you another more relevant example. This is not actually a real person, but is a typical scenario.

Jane had not had any major health problems – just a couple of painful bouts of cystitis (bladder infection) in her twenties. She is a person who likes to do things well and often leaves little time to relax.

Over a period of time she noticed that she needed to urinate more and more often, up to 20 times a day. She experienced a strong feeling of the need to pass water, which went away for a while after she had done so, but soon came back. In an attempt to go to the toilet less often, she began to drink less fluid, thinking that then there would be less need to go. She worried that if she didn't urinate when she felt the first urge, the discomfort would just get worse or she might have been incontinent. These worries led her to urinate when she could, 'just in case'. For example, she would always go two or three times before going to work or going out. She also noticed that when she was feeling stressed or upset, her bladder was even more sensitive. She worried about her bladder and what people would think of her trips to the toilet every 20 minutes. She avoided being away from a toilet for too long and often stayed in.

After Jane was given some general information and advice about slowly reducing how often she urinates and increasing her fluids again to encourage the bladder to work normally and practising some relaxation techniques, Jane has reduced her frequency of passing water to a 'normal' level and no longer feels discomfort or worries about her bladder ruling her life.

The rest of this book is about increasing your sense of control over your particular bladder difficulties. The first step is always understanding the problem, so the first three chapters are aimed at giving you the knowledge you need to understand the symptoms you are experiencing – what causes them and what kinds of medical tests and procedures you may encounter.

Chapter 4 is about the many kinds of physical and emotional factors that can affect how your bladder works.

Chapters 5, 6 and 7 are about changing what you do to improve your symptoms as much as possible.

As your bladder is only as healthy as the rest of you, general lifestyle and health issues that may help are discussed in Chapter 8.

Chapters 9 and 10 are particularly aimed at recognizing and modifying the effects of stress and worry on your bladder problems. Although it is common knowledge that the bladder is extremely sensitive to any worry or anxiety, particularly if that anxiety is about the bladder itself, this is hardly ever an area where people receive help.

Summary

Millions of people have irritable bladder problems. The main problems are urgency and frequency of passing water. There is enormous variety in the way people react and, hence, cope with these bladder problems and it can be particularly difficult to discuss them.

Whatever your particular problems are and however you are dealing with them, this book can help you to increase your sense of knowledge and control, improve your symptoms and cope successfully with them.

1

What are your symptoms?

The very first, and most important, step in learning to better cope with your bladder problems is to know exactly how things are at the moment. This may sound a little strange, you may think you know what your difficulties are already, but we need to be specific and clear right from the start for a number of reasons. First, this will enable you, in a few weeks' or months' time, to look at how things have improved and this can be a great motivator to carry on making changes. Second, because the problems you are experiencing may upset you, there will be an understandable temptation to either underplay the problem (if I ignore it will go away) or feel overwhelmed by it (things are so bad there is nothing I can do). Neither of these views will help you cope with or control your symptoms in the long term. Being as objective as possible can help. Third, keeping a record of your symptoms is an essential part of planning the right programme for yourself. Lastly, if you have a good idea of what your symptoms are, then it may help any medical staff you consult to understand and treat the problem in the best way.

Right, so the first step is to be clear about the nature of the beast! Irritable bladder symptoms are frequent bladder emptying, feelings of urgency to pass water and sometimes discomfort. Incontinence sufferers often experience these problems to a greater or lesser extent. Urgency and frequency are by no means always linked with incontinence, although sufferers may fear this happening. For this reason, incontinence is also discussed in the book. Other symptoms can include bowel problems, abdominal aches and headaches.

So, bladder symptoms are generally of three main types – frequency and urgency of urination, discomfort and incontinence. Let's consider each of these in more detail and then discuss ways in which you can monitor your own symptoms.

Frequency and urgency

Most bladder problems are accompanied by some change in the frequency of urination. That is, how often you visit the toilet to empty

7

your bladder. Usually there is also a change in the feeling of the bladder, which leads to a change in a person's behaviour. Urgency or 'urge' is a sudden, strong feeling of the need to empty the bladder. So, if someone visits the toilet more often, this is because of an increased feeling of the urge to urinate. If someone visits the toilet less often, then there may be a reduced feeling or urge to urinate.

What is 'normal' in terms of frequency of bladder emptying? As with all human experience and functioning, everyone is different in how often they need to empty their bladders. Research has found that, for most people, frequency is about six or seven times a day, but anywhere between four and ten times a day can be perfectly 'normal', in the sense that the person is healthy and not concerned about their bladder and there have been no unexplained changes.

What is normal also depends on a large number of other things that can affect the bladder. For example, the amount and type of fluid you drink, the temperature, how active you are and your age, to name a few. Some of these factors and others will be discussed in greater detail in Chapters 2 and 4. It is unusual, though, to have to get up more than once a night to visit the toilet. Try to work out how often you usually visit the toilet each day (don't worry if it seems a lot, it's important to be honest with yourself). Do you have to get out of bed at night to empty your bladder? If so how many times? What is it that leads to you emptying your bladder? Is it the urge to urinate or do you often go out of habit or 'just in case'? Start to think about this last question next time you go.

Very frequent urination can interfere enormously with everyday life and can become a source of great worry and embarrassment. This can develop to the extent that it becomes a major concern and life is planned around the problem. In fact, it is usually not just the *number* of times the person has to urinate that is the central concern, but the uncomfortable feeling of the need and urgency to urinate and the worrying about the problem. Again, there is a great deal of variation in the amount and kind of urgency or discomfort that people experience and a range of possible causes.

Pain and discomfort

Sometimes people's major concern about their bladder is to do with changes in feeling. As we all know, the feeling of urgency or needing to empty the bladder can be rather uncomfortable and also very

8

preoccupying, making it difficult to think about anything else. If you are emptying the bladder frequently, it is likely that you are also suffering some discomfort in terms of urgency. Many people find their discomfort is temporarily relieved by emptying the bladder. Is this true for you? Often people have fears about the discomfort getting worse and use bladder emptying to prevent this. Of course this only works in the short term, as, in the long term, you are training your bladder to cope with smaller volumes of urine and to become more sensitive. I will discuss this kind of 'vicious circle' more in Chapter 4.

There are also other kinds of discomfort associated with bladder problems. Some people experience more continual discomfort and aching around the groin and even backaches. For some, passing water itself is painful.

Do you suffer from any discomfort or pain? If so, where do you experience the feelings? What is the pattern of the discomfort? Does it come and go? If so, what makes it worse or better? Spend a few moments thinking about this.

Incontinence

As we have discussed, losing urine involuntarily is a very common problem, although by no means everyone with irritable bladder will experience this. Yet again, there is enormous variation when it comes to people's experiences of incontinence. I would certainly defy any woman to say that they have never laughed or coughed so hard that they have lost some urine (hence the phrase 'I nearly wet myself'!) I will describe how and why this occurs in the next chapter.

At the other end of the spectrum, a person may have to deal with being continually wet or with losing a large amount of urine in one go. The *pattern* of urine loss is important in determining the kind of problem you have and how to treat it. Begin to consider your own individual pattern.

If you ever loose urine, is it linked with particular events, such as coughing or certain movements? Is it worse when you are feeling stressed? How many times a day/week is it happening? Does it follow a strong and sudden urge to urinate? Are there certain activities and situations that you avoid for fear of being incontinent?

Worry and distress

I said at the beginning of this chapter that there are *three* main groups of symptoms associated with bladder problems – frequency, discomfort and incontinence. We have begun to consider what these are and whether they are a problem for you. There is, however, still a huge piece of the picture missing that is rarely talked about. This can be the key to gaining control over your symptoms. This is how you *feel* about what is happening. You will remember from the Introduction how thoughts and feelings about symptoms can affect how you deal with them and the outcome.

We know that having bladder problems can be stressful. In fact, this can become a major problem in itself. This upset can help to keep the difficulties going since the bladder is extremely sensitive to stress. Everyone who has been anxious (for example, before taking a driving test) will testify to the effect this has on the bladder.

Are stress and worry playing a major part in your bladder problems? Is the problem on your mind most of the time? Do you feel that it rules your life? Have you enjoyed activities less as a result or do you routinely avoid situations? Do you have difficulty sleeping? Have you told anyone how you feel? This is something I will return to throughout the book.

What next?

Having introduced the main symptoms of irritable bladder syndrome, there are three important steps to think about before beginning any programme to improve your symptoms.

The first step

I have started you thinking about the kinds of symptoms you have and how they might be affecting you. As I have said, one of the keys to success will be understanding your difficulties and making changes. I am going to ask you to keep records of your symptoms, to understand the possible mechanisms involved and make changes in what you do. All this requires a good deal of hard work if you are going to be successful – just reading this book will not change things. However, if it *does* change what you do and how you feel, you are on the road to coping successfully. Remember the old saying, a journey of a thousand miles begins with the first step.

One of the things that can hold you back is the way you see your problem.

Ways of thinking that will hold you back
- thinking that the problem is your fault
- thinking that nothing can be done
- thinking that people will judge you harshly
- thinking that you could not cope with the embarrassment of going to the doctor
- thinking that the problem makes you less of a person
- thinking of all the things you can't do
- blaming yourself for your bladder problems.

Ask yourself
- If my best friend told me they had a bladder problem, would I think less of them?
- What would I advise them to do?
- Would I feel the same if the problem was, for example, a broken leg?
- What action would I take for any other physical problem?
- What can I do?

Ways of thinking that encourage you
- wanting to understand what the problem is
- wanting to make changes that will improve the situation
- being able to tell someone honestly how you feel about the problem
- getting the help you need
- doing what you can
- telling yourself how well you are doing.

The second step

The second step is to begin keeping records for yourself. Decide whether or not you have difficulty with frequency, pain or incontinence, or any combination of these, so that you know what to record.

Keep a diary sheet, like the one below (Figure 1.1), for a week to give you a 'baseline' to work from. This will give you time to read through the rest of the book and prepare yourself for any changes you decide to make. I have given you two columns for each day and divided each day into hours. You might wish to make your own version. For example, if you want to record frequency, pain and incontinence, you might want three columns, if you get up a lot at night, you might want to break that time down in more detail.

WHAT ARE YOUR SYMPTOMS?

	Sun		Mon		Tues		Wed		Thur		Fri		Sat	
6 am														
7 am														
8 am														
9 am														
10 am														
11 am														
12 am														
1 pm														
2 pm														
3 pm														
4 pm														
5 pm														
6 pm														
7 pm														
8 pm														
9 pm														
10 pm														
11 pm														
12 pm														
1–5 am														

Figure 1.1 A weekly diary sheet for monitoring bladder symptoms

12

Here's what to do. To record *frequency* of bladder emptying, simply tick in the appropriate box. So, if you wake up at 8 am on Monday morning and go straight to the toilet, put a tick in that box. Of course, you may go more than once in that hour, in which case, put more than one tick in the box. Every time you empty your bladder, record it on the sheet.

To record *discomfort*, rate how bad it is from one to ten, where one is no discomfort and ten is very severe discomfort or pain.

To record *incontinence*, put a cross in the appropriate box for the time when the incontinence occurs and a rating of small (s), medium (m) or large (l) for the amount lost. Small is just a little, making you damp, medium is a moderate amount, say an egg cupful, and large is a significant amount or when your bladder has emptied completely.

The third step

We all need support and help in dealing with our problems and to motivate us to make the changes necessary to gain control over them. If you take the decision to make changes, then also decide to find yourself a helper.

Who you choose will depend on you and your circumstances. You might like to ask someone in the family or a close friend. If this seems difficult, you might find it easier to talk to someone more detached, such as a doctor or a practice nurse. If you have not discussed your difficulties with anyone, it may be a huge relief to do so and I am sure you will be surprised how supportive people are. Of course, you won't want too many people to know, confidentiality is also important, so choose someone that you trust. Just think about who you could talk to for the time being and, as you continue to read the book and decide which bits apply to you, it will become clearer how they could be supportive.

I have said that people often avoid going to the doctor with bladder problems. They may be too embarrassed or feel that the problem is too trivial or think that nothing can be done. The bladder is a part of the body like any other and the doctor will try to put you at ease. There are effective treatments for most bladder problems, so the long-term gain of visiting the doctor in terms of the quality of your life should be weighed against your understandable short-term fears.

Make an appointment to see your doctor if

- you have never had your bladder difficulties assessed by a doctor
- you notice any sudden changes in bladder function
- you have any other symptoms, even if they seem unrelated to the bladder
- you notice blood in your urine
- passing urine is painful
- you feel the need to empty your bladder again immediately after you have just emptied it
- it is difficult to urinate or the flow is slow or interrupted
- you have continuous incontinence
- you are very distressed by your bladder problems.

The medical tests, treatments and terminology that you may come across are discussed in Chapter 3.

Summary

I have started to describe the kinds of bladder symptoms that are commonly experienced and, hopefully, you will begin to keep clear records of your own particular symptoms. The three main kinds of bladder symptoms were introduced – frequency and urgency, discomfort and incontinence. Keeping a diary will give you a good idea about your own symptoms. Making changes can be hard work, so make sure you have the support you need.

2

Causes of bladder symptoms

Generally, we get concerned when we notice some changes in how our bodies are working. These changes or 'symptoms' can be due to a number of factors. Understanding your symptoms will hopefully lessen your concern and make it clearer how to cope with them. Not all symptoms, particularly those of irritable bladder, are necessarily caused by a disease process or 'medical' condition. Remember that the symptoms of irritable bladder problems are a feeling of needing to urinate (urgency), urinating more often than normal (frequency), sometimes feelings of discomfort and, for some people, incontinence. However, some of these same symptoms can occur in other conditions, which I will also discuss.

In this chapter I shall begin by describing normal bladder functioning. It is then easy to describe how the symptoms of frequency/urgency, discomfort and incontinence can arise. I will say what conditions groups of symptoms indicate and discuss the current thinking about mechanisms and causes of bladder problems. Tests and treatments are discussed in the next chapter.

Normal bladder functioning

At its most basic level, the bladder is a collecting point for urine that it stores until there is a convenient place to urinate. Urine is produced by the kidneys and travels down the ureters into the bladder (see Figure 2.1). The kidneys serve the function of helping the body to regulate the amount of water and salt in the body. So, if you drink a lot of water, your kidneys will filter off the excess, this process takes around one to two hours. If you drink very little or are losing water in other ways, for example sweating on a hot day, then less, more concentrated urine is produced.

As more urine enters, the wall of the bladder, which is actually a muscle, relaxes to allow more to be stored. Most adult bladders do not need to be emptied more than every two to four hours and can store around 400 to 600 ml (14 fl oz to 1 pint) of urine. Fill a measuring jug with water to see just how much this is. Try also collecting your urine on a couple of occasions into a plastic measuring jug to see how much

15

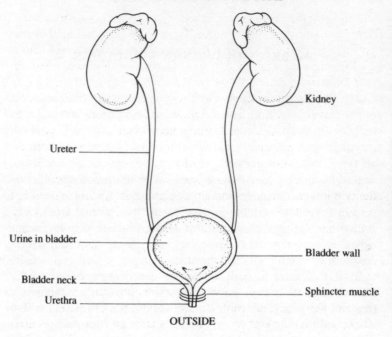

Figure 2.1 Urine produced in the kidneys travels down the ureters to the bladder

you can typically hold in your bladder. Urine is normally sterile and odourless as it leaves the body, so all you have to do is give the jug a good rinse afterwards.

As the bladder relaxes on filling, the muscle at the bottom of the bladder contracts to keep the urethra shut so that the urine is contained. It's rather like a balloon filled with water that is being pinched at the bottom to keep the water in. It's also rather like your stomach in that, at a certain point, you will become aware of a feeling of fullness. In the case of the bladder filling, you will then feel the urge to urinate.

The bladder-empting process is the opposite of the filling one. So, on filling, the bladder relaxes and the opening contracts, while, on emptying, the bladder contracts, to expel the urine, and the sphincter muscle at the opening relaxes to allow the urine to flow out.

The actual control of this process is rather complicated. What is interesting is that, like some other bodily functions, bladder control is a combination of automatic (reflex) and voluntary responses.

16

Reflex responses are not under voluntary control. So, for example, if the doctor taps your knee in the right way, your leg jerks out of your control, and if air is puffed at your eye, you will blink. In babies, bladder emptying is purely reflexive. The bladder fills with urine and, at a certain state of fullness, the nerves send a message that allows the bladder to contract. It is only later in development that the ability to control this reflex voluntarily is gained, and urination can be delayed until convenient. Other bodily functions that are also part automatic reflex and part voluntary are breathing and swallowing. Both are processes that work perfectly naturally, but can also come under conscious control. Have you noticed how once you start paying attention to your breathing that this seems to alter it and make it feel unnatural? Could this also apply to your bladder problem? These kinds of bodily processes are often the ones affected by emotional factors, such as worry. For example, worry can lead to fast, shallow breathing and a feeling of tightness in the throat and also the need to urinate. I shall discuss these issues in greater depth in Chapter 4.

There are just a few more things about bladder functioning that are relevant to us. They are to do with the importance of the pelvic floor muscles (see Figure 2.2) and differences between men and women.

The pelvic floor muscles play an important role in bladder

Figure 2.2 The position of the pelvic floor muscle

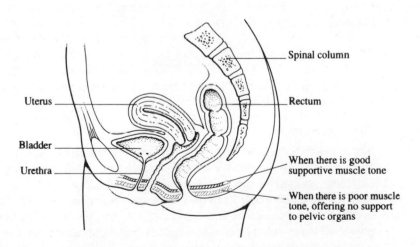

Spinal column

Uterus

Rectum

Bladder

Urethra

When there is good
supportive muscle tone

When there is poor muscle
tone, offering no support
to pelvic organs

functioning. For one thing, they help the opening of the bladder to stay shut as it fills with urine. The pelvic floor muscles support the pelvic organs – the bladder, the uterus, in women, and the bowel – in a kind of sling. If the muscles are damaged in anyway, for example, by childbirth or surgery, then this can lead to bowel and bladder problems, such as constipation and incontinence. Similarly, if the muscles are overtensed, perhaps due to habit or in response to pain, then difficulties in passing water can ensue. If you are female, next time you empty your bladder, try to stop the stream in midflow. The muscles you use to do this are the pelvic floor muscles. Did you feel them tighten up? If it was difficult to stop the flow, then it may be that your pelvic floor muscles are rather weak. Do not repeat this 'stop' exercise too often as it is important that you always empty your bladder completely.

The role of the pelvic floor muscles is often of particular importance for women with bladder problems, but men, too, have pelvic floor muscles that can be damaged by prostate surgery, for example. In terms of passing water, women tend to rely, to some extent, on raising abdominal pressure by bearing down to squeeze the bladder. There is rather more emphasis in men on the muscle at the neck of the bladder. This means men can more easily 'shut off' the flow of urine once it is underway using this muscle than women. But also, conversely, some men have difficulty *starting* bladder emptying, especially when they are anxious.

So, now we know a little about the normal functioning of the bladder, what can go wrong?

Incontinence

There are various kinds of incontinence and the causes can be quite varied. Let us now look at the different kinds.

Stress incontinence

Stress incontinence is to do with physical rather than emotinal stress. Urine is lost on physical exertion, such as coughing, sneezing, laughing, jumping or running. Essentially, what happens is that the muscles which normally keep the bladder opening closed have been unable to do so due to the increased pressure (stress) caused by the physical movement. Try coughing gently and, whether you experience this problem or not, you will be able to feel the strain on the

18

abdomen and pelvic floor that can cause a loss of urine. Usually, the amount of urine lost due to stress incontinence is small, but is, of course, inconvenient and people who experience it may well avoid certain activities, such as sports and other physical activities.

Stress incontinence can be caused by a weakness either at the level of the actual sphincter (the ring of muscle that closes the urethra) or of the pelvic floor muscles (which support the bladder). Problems can be triggered by trauma to the area, the most typical examples being childbirth and surgery.

If you lose urine immediately on exertion, you probably have stress incontinence. Pluck up the courage to speak to your doctor about it if you have not already done so. The most common treatment for stress incontinence is pelvic floor exercises, which are often entirely effective (these are described in Chapter 7). Surgery may be recommended for very severe cases, but only when more conservative treatment efforts have failed.

Overflow incontinence

Overflow incontinence is like the opposite to stress incontinence. Rather than urine escaping too easily from the bladder, the bladder-emptying mechanism is obstructed in some way. Once the bladder is full, the high pressure means that urine is forced out in a steady dribble.

Enlargement of the prostate gland in men can obstruct bladder emptying. The other possibility is that there is an abnormal hole somewhere that allows urine to escape.

Obviously, you need medical attention for these symptoms and so you should see your doctor.

Irritable bladder problems

The various problems described below are those I generally term 'irritable bladder', which are different to those where there is some clear cause, such as infection. This is because they all involve the symptoms of frequency and urgency described earlier and are often made worse by stress.

Urge incontinence

Urge incontinence is more to do with the behaviour of the bladder muscle itself than either stress or overflow incontinence. This kind of incontinence always involves a strong sensation of the urge to empty the bladder accompanied by a loss of urine.

One cause of urge incontinence is the bladder muscle contracting, as it would to empty the bladder, despite the person's attempts to inhibit this. This is more correctly called 'motor urge incontinence'. The amount of urine lost is typically large – usually the contents of the bladder. This kind of 'bladder instability', as it is also known, can only be properly assessed by the appropriate specialist tests. Sometimes the bladder contractions can be triggered by physical events, such as coughing, but there is a delay between the event and the incontinence. This kind of incontinence is also associated with bedwetting, or 'enuresis', which is when the bladder-voiding reflex occurs during sleep.

Bladder instability can also be caused by obstructions to emptying, such as an enlarged prostate gland or bladder stones.

If you have these kinds of symptoms, make an appoitment with your doctor to discuss them before embarking on a self-help programme. Often, there is no obvious physical reason for the bladder contracting in this way. The bladder is affected by many different factors, not all of them physical, however (see also Chapter 4).

Sometimes, there can be incontinence and a sense of urgency without there being actual bladder contractions and this is more correctly termed 'sensory urge incontinence'. Usually, the amount of urine lost is little.

Motor and sensory urge incontinence, including bedwetting, tend to respond well to bladder-training procedures, which are described in Chapter 7.

Urgency and frequency

Urgency and frequency are obviously associated with the urge incontinence problems described above. However, they also often exist on their own, without incontinence. This syndrome has many names and many proposed causes, but the essential elements are those of a bladder that is sensitive, often uncomfortable in terms of the feeling of urgency, compelling its owner to visit the toilet frequently and lead a life that is ruled by their bladder problems.

Ironically, sufferers are rarely incontinent, but often live in fear of this possibility and restrict their lifestyles accordingly. If you follow the procedures described in this book, you will have an excellent chance of overcoming your difficulties in time.

There can be underlying factors associated with chronic urgency and frequency, such as a low-grade infection of some kind, so this possibility should be excluded by having the correct medical tests and treatment before doing anything else.

Pain and discomfort

When urgency and frequency, and possibly incontinence, are associated with pain, particularly if there is pain on passing urine, then you probably have an infection. You should, of course, seek out the appropriate treatment.

Most people have heard of cystitis and it is often used to describe bladder infections. Usually, such infections are simply caused by bacteria from the bowel entering the bladder, but occasionally it may be that there are additional problems, such as bladder stones.

Cystitis is far more common in women than men, with 10 per cent of women thought to suffer from it each year. This is because in women the urethra is close to the anus and then bacteria only have a short distance to travel up the urethra to the bladder. Cystitis can also be caused by other organisms, however. Infections are usually fairly short-lived and can sometimes be overcome by drinking copious amounts of water to dilute the bacteria. You should always consult your doctor if the symptoms last more than a day, if you have blood in your urine and if there are any other symptoms, such as fever.

There is evidence to suggest that some women are prone to suffering recurrent bouts of cystitis. This can be very stressful and debilitating. Your doctor should be able to help you find the most appropriate treatment and there are a number of self-help procedures that are extremely effective. The key points are to always drink plenty of bland fluid and empty your bladder every two hours, and always wash the vaginal area and empty the bladder before and after sex. Also, follow the general advice given in Chapters 5 to 10 of this book. There are some excellent self-help books on the topic of recurrent cystitis – see the Further reading section at the end of the book.

If you suffer from urgency, frequency and pain all the time, it is likely that you have been told you have interstitial cystitis. This is an inflammation of the lining of the bladder, rather like having a stomach ulcer.

There is some disagreement about the cause of this syndrome and it is likely that there are a number of different ones. Some researchers argue that the cause is often to do with some infection, others that there is a disorder of the immune system.

Mild symptoms can be helped by the procedures described in Chapters 5 to 10 in this book, while those who are suffering severe symptoms are sometimes offered surgery.

Sometimes bladder problems are associated not with the acute, sharp pain of an infection, but with chronic aches and discomfort that come and go. Incontinence and irritable bladder are associated with a range of other symptoms. Sufferers often also have irritable bowel problems, recurrent headaches and backaches, as well as discomfort in the lower abdomen.

If physical causes for these symptoms have been eliminated, then it is likely that they are stress related. Many of my patients are initially mystified at how stress can cause pain. One of the first things that happens when you feel stressed is that you tense up. Different people tend to get tense in different ways. Some people suffer from headaches because their neck muscles are all tensed up. If you are tense about your bladder, it makes sense that you will tense up around the pelvic area, which can lead to aches and pains over time. If you doubt that muscle tension can cause pain, think of the agony of cramp, which is just that! If you think this may apply to you, then read Chapters 5 to 10 carefully.

Summary

I have covered some basic information about how the bladder works and what can go wrong. I hope that this has helped you to make more sense of the symptoms that you have been suffering. In the next chapter, I will describe the kinds of medical tests that are currently available and common treatments.

3

Medical tests, treatments
and terms

I mentioned earlier that you should make an appointment to see your doctor if you have not already done so. I know that many people are reluctant to visit the doctor and put off doing so. When people are asked why this is, particularly incontinence sufferers, they give a number of reasons. Often people are unclear whether or not bladder difficulties represent a legitimate medical concern. They feel that their problems are an almost inevitable price to pay for getting older, having babies or whatever. They may feel a great sense of embarrassment at the thought of discussing these problems and be unsure of the reception that they will receive. It is as if people hide such difficulties as a way of coping, that if they don't talk about them, they're not really a problem. Often even close friends and family are unaware of the extent of someone's difficulties.

Are you putting off getting the appropriate help and support for these kinds of reasons? The situation is unlikely to improve if you ignore it. In fact, quite the opposite can be true and, anyway, why put up with troublesome symptoms if effective help is easily available? I will try to give you a good idea of the kinds of things to expect when you visit your doctor – what they will ask you, the kinds of examinations and tests they may undertake and the treatments they might suggest. I will also describe the kinds of investigations you might experience if you are referred to a urology clinic at the hospital and the kinds of treatments they may offer you. At the back of the book is an alphabetical list of some of the medical terms you might come across.

Going to see your doctor

The first step is to make your appointment. Consider ways to make this as easy on yourself as possible. Allow adequate time, take a friend along to wait with you if this helps or perhaps a good book or magazine to distract you.

If you have been putting off going because, for example, your doctor is male and you would rather see a woman (or the opposite perhaps if you are a man), you have a number of options. All doctors see a large number of people with bladder problems, so, hopefully, male and female doctors should be equally sympathetic. If you are registered with a group practice, then ask to see the person you would feel most at ease with. There is no need to tell the receptionist why you are making this request. All medical conversations are confidential. Remember, you are probably a hundred-fold more uncomfortable about this consultation than your doctor. For them it is routine. If you are particularly anxious, it might be worth mentioning this to them so that they can do their best to put you at your ease.

Once you are with your doctor, mention any specific fears you might have, such as anxieties about needles or blood. If these are a problem for you, you may need help to tackle them. Phobias like these can be easily conquered given the correct help and support. Ask your doctor to recommend someone who can help you or ask them to refer you to the local clinical psychology service. If you choose an independent practitioner, check that they have appropriate qualifications (anyone can call themselves a psychologist, even if they have had no proper training). In my work I have seen many people overcome these kinds of fears in a matter of weeks and they feel much more confident because of this.

Your doctor will find it very helpful if you have been keeping a diary of your symptoms. The pattern of your symptoms will help them to decide on the next steps to take. So, take your completed copy of the diary on page 12 with you when you go.

You will probably also be asked to provide a specimen of urine. If you would rather take this with you than have to produce one at the surgery, then either call into the surgery before the appointment to pick up a specimen bottle or use any small, clean, watertight container. You only need to collect about an egg cupful, but make sure the sample is a 'midstream' one. This means you need to start urinating, stop the flow, if you can, and then collect your sample in the middle of the flow. As you can imagine, this can be a bit tricky!

The specimen is needed to check whether or not there is any infection in the bladder. The results of the test will take a few days to come back. The doctor may also test whether there is sugar in the urine to check for diabetes and may also test for blood in the urine. They can usually do these latter two tests at the surgery.

Write down the details of all medications that you take, especially if you are not seeing your usual doctor.

Hopefully, if you have kept a diary and been thinking about your symptoms, you will easily be able to answer questions about frequency, urgency and discomfort and incontinence.

Your doctor may also ask questions about other aspects of your health and is likely to examine you. You may have your blood pressure taken or the doctor may want to do a blood test to check the levels of certain hormones and other substances in your system. In terms of physical examinations, the doctor will probably want to feel your abdomen to check for any abnormalities. They will also want to do a rectal and vaginal examination to check, by looking and feeling, for abnormalities, constipation or infection. This is probably the most anxiety provoking part of the procedure, but it is essential if the doctor is to arrive at the right conclusions and to eliminate the possibility of there being any structural problems. Try to relax if you feel uptight at this stage. Remember that you are free to ask the doctor to explain fully what they are doing, to stop at any time, particularly if you feel any discomfort, and to take someone in with you if you want to.

Treatment

The doctor may ask to see you again to discuss the results of the tests, may refer you to a hospital clinic or may, at this stage, recommend some form of treatment. The doctor may refer you to a physiotherapist for pelvic floor exercises if they think that pelvic floor weakness is contributing to your difficulties (these are discussed in more detail in Chapter 7).

The next possibility is that you may be prescribed some medication, in the form of tablets. If you have urge incontinence, you may be prescribed oxybutynin. The effect of this is to reduce uncontrolled bladder contractions. A similar drug you may be prescribed is imipramine, which needs to be taken for about a week if you are to notice a therapeutic effect.

Drugs act on the whole body, of course, and often there are some side-effects of treatment. For treatment to be effective, the drugs have to be taken in dosages at which you are almost certain to notice other effects. These can include a dry mouth, blurred vision, increased heart rate and flushing. You may also feel drowsy, dizzy, nauseous or get constipated. Different people are affected differently by side-effects and they tend to improve over time. Some people find the treatment difficult to tolerate, so don't worry if this applies to you, keep a note of any symptoms and report back to your doctor. If you develop a difficulty in passing urine, contact your doctor immediately.

Although these drugs are not addictive, they are acting on your nervous system. Medication may help symptoms and for some people will sort the problem out, but, in the long term, of course, you will need to cope without it. If you embark on a self-help programme, ask your doctor if you can try to solve the problem without drugs in the first instance as this will allow your bladder to be trained under normal circumstances and you will have a better chance of long-term success.

Sometimes muscle relaxants or tranquillizers are prescribed for problems such as sensory urgency. Again, this may help in the short term, but these drugs are addictive and so are not for long-term use. Why not try the programme in this book or ask what advice the doctor can give, other than drug therapy? Always make sure you understand (and write down if you are likely to forget) the name of the drug being prescribed, its mode of action – for example, if it is a tranquillizer – and likely side-effects.

Other forms of medication may include antibiotic or antifungal agents, if you have an infection, or hormone replacement therapy if your doctor thinks this may help your symptoms. Remember that finding the right treatment is a collaborative venture. You need to give the doctor accurate information and feedback about whether or not the treatment prescribed is working. You should be able to discuss the alternatives and it may be that drug therapy is not appropriate. Your doctor may give you some general advice, like that in this book, about bladder training, fluid intake and diet, and these approaches can be combined with medication.

Going to the hospital

If you are referred to a urology, genito-urinary, or urological gynaecology urology department of a hospital, you may undergo some other tests. Again, take along your diary, a note of any medication and be prepared to provide a specimen of urine – that is, don't empty your bladder before you see the doctor.

The following description will give you a general idea of what goes on, but, obviously, each department will vary one from the other. You should be given a full explanation of any procedures by the clinic staff, but, if in doubt, ask.

Some departments will have a portable ultrasound machine (like the ones used for showing mothers-to-be a scan of their unborn babies), which will allow the doctor to see the bladder and may show up certain problems, such as bladder stones.

If blood was found in your urine then you may be asked to come for a cystoscopy. This is a fairly simple out-patient procedure where a minute camera within a fine tube is inserted into the bladder so that the doctor can see if there is any abnormality, such as inflammation or growth.

Urodynamic studies (or cystometry) involves a series of tests to assess the behaviour of the bladder on filling and emptying. These are usually recommended when there is a mixture of symptoms, an operation is being considered or previous treatment has not been effective. You are usually asked to attend with a full bladder and to pass urine, in private, into a commode that records the amount of urine you pass and the rate at which it flows.

The next stage is completed while you are lying down. A small tube or catheter is passed into the bladder, which will be used to fill the bladder. Another fine tube will also be inserted that will measure pressure and a further similar one is inserted into the rectum to measure abdominal pressure. Although you may feel some discomfort while the catheters are being put into place, this is usually mild and wears off quickly.

The bladder is then slowly filled with fluid and you will be asked to indicate when you first get the desire to empty your bladder and then when you feel that you really must go. The filling tube is then removed and you will be asked to stand and move or cough.

Finally, you will be asked to empty your bladder so that volume and flow can again be recorded. After the pressure recorders are removed, the procedure is complete.

I know this test doesn't sound too pleasant, but it does allow a proper assessment to be made of how well the bladder is functioning, and staff will explain each part of the procedure. Again, if you are feeling tense, try to practise some relaxation techniques in advance of the appointment and put them into use on the day. Generally, you will know beforehand that you will have a certain procedure and will be given all the information you need to prepare yourself for it.

Treatment

The hospital doctor may recommend the same kind of drug treatment your doctor might offer (see the beginning of this chapter), physiotherapy if there is weakness of the pelvic floor muscles, an intensive course of bladder retraining or surgery. Bladder retraining may take place either on an out- or in-patient basis and is fundamentally an intensive course to re-educate the bladder (the basics of bladder retraining are considered in Chapter 7). Surgery may involve repairing the pelvic floor, correcting a prolapse of any of the pelvic organs or a weakness in the bladder neck. Sometimes there is an obstruction in the bladder or urethra that needs to be removed, or, in males, an enlarged prostate gland may be hindering bladder emptying and so it needs to be removed. Also, if less invasive treatments for an unstable bladder have failed, then surgery is sometimes recommended. This might involve interrupting the nerve supply to the bladder wall or inserting a piece of bowel material into the bladder wall to make it larger. All surgery has potential drawbacks and you should be sure you understand what is being recommended, what the alternatives and risks are and why the surgery is considered to be the next step rather than anything else. It is, of course, only a small minority of people who will end up at the hospital or having any kind of surgery.

Two final procedures that are now more rarely used for bladder problems and are sometimes recommended for sensory urgency or interstitial cystitis are the stretching of the urethra or the bladder. The bladder is stretched by overfilling it with fluid for a long period. There are risks associated with such procedures and it is not clear whether or not people benefit from them in the long term. Again, make sure you know the pros and cons of any procedure that is recommended.

What next?

If you have consulted your doctor and have a good idea about your particular difficulties, then, hopefully, you will have more idea of how to overcome them. You may have been given certain treatments and advice and can enhance these by following the appropriate sections of the programme of bladder training, pelvic floor exercises and general lifestyle changes that I will go on to describe.

4

Physical and emotional factors
and the bladder

The bladder is a sensitive beast! Its functioning can be influenced by a whole range of factors. Fortunately, most of these factors are directly under your control, or can be improved by taking the appropriate action. As with most things in life, it is usually the case that there is no single, simple 'cause' of bladder difficulties that can be put right immediately by, for example, the doctor. Usually, such difficulties worsen over time, perhaps for a number of reasons, and require a 'multifactorial' approach. I hope to describe as many things that can affect bladder functioning as possible, and to illustrate how these factors can come to interact so that symptoms are maintained over time.

Diet

The idea that your diet can influence your bladder may seem slightly odd. It is really, though, the *effects* of your diet that are important. So, for example, chronic constipation can result from your diet and may cause problems. Remember that the rectum and the bladder are close together and are both supported by the pelvic floor muscles. Straining to go to the toilet stretches and weakens these muscles. If constipation is a constant problem for you, then it may be advisable to seek some medical help. If it is occasionally a problem, then it is a good idea to pay special attention to your diet. The most common causes of constipation are a lack of fibre in the diet, not enough exercise, ignoring the need to empty the bowel and certain drugs. Drinking too little fluid may also be a factor.

The other possible influence your diet may have is that being overweight can adversely affect your bladder. Remember that the bladder is supported by the pelvic floor, which can be overworked if you are overweight.

Some say that certain kinds of foods, such as very spicy ones, can influence the bladder. It is probably advisable to avoid very salty foods as too much salt can be dehydrating. In general, try to follow the advice given in Chapter 8.

Drinks

It's probably a little easier to see the connection between what you drink and your bladder – the link is more direct. Most of us don't drink enough fluid and don't drink the right things, but rectifying this situation is especially important if you have a bladder problem.

Resist the temptation to reduce your intake of fluids as a way of coping with frequency and urgency at all costs. This is not good for your health in general and merely trains your bladder to cope with less and less fluid over time; that is, you are making it *more* sensitive. The recommended daily intake of fluid is about eight to ten glasses of water a day, or around 1.75 litres (3 pints). This seems a lot I know, but is easiest if you increase your intake slowly. Many of the people I have seen who have managed this had reduced their intake to small sips, or about *one* glass a day.

The other major factor is *what* you drink. The most important thing to avoid is caffeine. This is a stimulant and has a very marked effect on bladder sensitivity! Other drinks to avoid in excess include alcohol – it is dehydrating – concentrated fruit juices and fizzy canned drinks, which are acidic.

As fluid intake is such an important issue, there is more detailed information and advice in Chapter 6.

Health

Other general health factors that may influence the bladder include coughing, lifting, medication and infections. Chronic coughing can be a problem because each time you cough you increase your abdominal pressure and the strain on the pelvic floor, in the long term, the bladder can be affected. Repeated heavy lifting can also put a strain on the pelvic floor. Try to avoid doing this or, otherwise, tighten the muscles consciously as you lift.

Certain kinds of drugs for other medical problems, such as diuretics (commonly known as 'water tablets') for high blood pressure, can alter bladder functioning. Bladder infections, such as cystitis, particulary recurrent attacks, can increase the sensitivity of the bladder in general. Just getting older can have an influence on the bladder and lead to other problems, such as having to get up at night.

A lot of bladder problems can be overcome or at least greatly relieved by following the self-help advice, particularly the pelvic floor exercises, which can improve things at any age. Regaining pelvic and abdominal muscle tone by means of appropriate excercises is a major step in the right direction.

Differences between women and men

For women there are certain events and influences in life that are important and may act as the starting point for bladder trouble. Pregnancy, childbirth and hysterectomy will all affect the bladder, even if this is only in the short term. Obviously they affect the abdomen and pelvic floor, where the bladder is located and supported. Hormonal changes may also be important, and, indeed, many women find that their bladder symptoms vary with their menstrual cycle. Also some women report symptoms when their menopause begins. The important message to repeat is that you should keep a diary of symptoms, consult your doctor where appropriate and follow the general advice in this book.

Although, on the whole, men have fewer bladder problems, it is not unusual for men to suffer incontinence and irritable bladder symptoms. Apart from the factors described immediately above, which relate to women, all the other causes of bladder problems mentioned so far, such as constipation, apply equally to men and women. The one particular physical factor that applies only to men, however, is the prostate gland. The prostate gland is at the base of the bladder and the urethra passes through it. If the prostate gland becomes enlarged, which often happens with age, the urethra becomes restricted and even blocked. The symptoms associated with this happening are:

- frequency
- discomfort on passing urine
- difficulty starting to pass urine and a slow stream
- dribbling incontinence
- having to get up at night to pass urine.

Your doctor will arrange for appropriate tests if it is thought that this is a problem for you and you may be advised to have a prostatectomy. This can be done in various ways and you may even only need a local anaesthetic. Remember to ask staff about any questions or concerns you have. Men commonly experience some bladder symptoms following the operation. Pelvic floor exercises may be helpful in improving bladder control and these are described in Chapter 7.

There is one other problem that can be a difficulty for men, although some women also suffer from it. This is difficulty in starting to urinate, or 'retention' of urine. This may only occur in particular circumstances. For example, quite a proportion of men find it difficult to urinate in front of others in a public toilet. Hardly surprising really!

This phenomenon is sometimes called 'bashful bladder'. It may be an occasional or mild problem, causing little disruption to everyday life, or it can develp over time until it becomes very restricting. I have talked to someone whose difficulties had generalized to include any public toilets, such that train journeys and an evening in the pub were a major source of anxiety.

Again, my advice is not to restrict your fluids as a way of coping with this. Learn a relaxation technique and talk yourself through it when you are having difficulty passing urine, taking the pressure off yourself to perform. If you cannot go after a minute or so, give up and try later – sometimes trying *not* to go will actually help!

Occasionally, difficulties in passing urine can be brought on by a severe shock or trauma, for example, the death of a loved one or experiencing an accident. This leads us into a discussion next of psychological factors that can affect the bladder.

Psychological factors

The bladder can often reflect the way we are feeling. One of the symptoms of anxiety and stress is an increased feeling of urgency, hence the frequent visits to the toilet before some big event. No one really understands the exact mechanism of this, but it is similar to the experience of 'butterflies in the stomach'. Our bodies are very much affected by our psychological state. Stress and anxiety are very individual things – no two people will experience the same event in the same way. Sometimes bladder problems date back to a time of 'acute' stress, such as a bereavement, or more prolonged 'strain' such as on-going marital, financial or work worries. Is this the case for you?

Whatever the initial 'triggers' of bladder problems may be, they can then be *maintained* by other factors. So, consider the following.

A person is under a lot of stress at work and home and the increased levels of anxiety lead to increased feelings of urgency and hence frequency of passing urine. Not making the link between the anxiety and these symptoms, the person begins to wonder about their cause. The nature of this wondering will depend on their personal experiences. So the woman whose mother had distressing problems of incontinence and confusion before she died, may fear a loss of control. The man who has an uncle with prostate trouble may fear physical illness. The sense that these people make of their difficulties then influences their actions. The woman might reduce her intake of fluids and increase the number of times she visits the toilet to (in her mind) reduce the risk of an 'accident'. Then she is likely to become very aware of any sensations of fullness in her bladder. Her anxiety, therefore, would not be allayed and her strategies would actually increase her bladder sensitivity over time, leading to more worry about symptoms and more attempts to control them. Can you see the vicious circle that develops? The man might visit the doctor and be referred for tests. He could then think that the doctor must think that there is something wrong. The tests would come back negative, but he would still have his symptoms. He could then think that he may have something 'worse' and ask for more tests. He might monitor his symptoms, worry about their significance and the anxiety would lead to more symptoms, confirming in his mind the presence of a serious problem. Another vicious circle is created.

Regardless now of how the work stress progresses in either case, the bladder symptoms are now under the influence of each person's thoughts and behaviour.

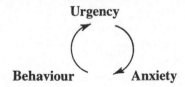

Figure 4.1 Anxiety helps set up a vicious circle that makes things worse

So anxiety, about other things or the symptoms themselves, can make bladder problems worse (see Figure 4.1). The signs of stress and anxiety are more fully explained in Chapter 9, but it is worth saying here that paying attention to the symptoms can make them worse. Often when I give talks on this topic, people will tell me afterwards that the more I talked about frequency, urgency and incontinence, the more they felt the need to go to the toilet. In fact, reading this book may have the initial effect of making you pay more attention to your bladder and hence experience more sensation. You can test out this idea yourself. Spend two minutes or so thinking about bladder sensations and concentrating on your bladder, then, on a scale of one to ten, rate how much of an urge to go to the toilet you felt while doing this. Then go off and read a column in the newspaper or a page in a book as if someone were going to ask you questions on it afterwards. Rate the urgency you felt again at the end of this time, without thinking about it too long. I hope you see the difference. Distraction techniques are described in Chapter 10 and they help to focus your attention away from the bladder so that the sensations are easier to cope with.

The bladder, therefore, is sensitive to anxiety and worry, to too much attention and it is 'suggestible' – if you think about going to the toilet you will want to go. It is also a creature of habit. If you always go to the toilet at a certain time, this trains the bladder and you may feel urgency in this situation whether the bladder is full or not. Sometimes these patterns are established in early childhood. My parents, and they were not alone, were in the habit of putting me on the toilet before we went out and running the tap to encourage me to go. To this day, for a lot of people, the sound of running water triggers the need to urinate! This is a process of learning links between events and it goes on throughout our lives. It is possible to unlearn these links by not succumbing to the urge. Each time you do this it becomes easier – honest.

Summary

There are various factors that can influence bladder functioning. I hope you can identify those that apply to you so that you can go on to make the kinds of changes that will reduce irritable bladder symptoms.

5

Pain and discomfort

Pain and discomfort are rather complex issues. There are a number of possible reasons for experiencing such difficulties, some of which I have already touched on. The other essential consideration is that the experience of pain and discomfort is never simply related to physical factors. Again, I shall explain and illustrate this point.

Have you ever injured yourself, even if it's only slightly, and not actually noticed until some time after the event? To take an example from my own experience, I remember going rock climbing (for the first and last time!) with some friends and being so focused on getting to the top of the cliff that I did not notice I had scraped some skin off the back of my hand until a few minutes after achieving my goal. I did not feel the pain at all during the climb. Under other circumstances – say, if I'd grazed my hand because I'd tripped over – I would have felt the pain immediately. And there are even more dramatic examples of this phenomenon, such as footballers and other athletes who break bones during the course of important matches and do not feel pain until after the game is over. This occurs because the feeling of pain is influenced by both messages from the nerves in the affected part of the body being sent up to the brain *and* by messages from the brain being sent back down to the site of the injury. The messages being sent *down* are related to your emotional and psychological state.

So, the implications of all this are that the same injury can feel different at different times. There is no simple one to one relationship between injury and the feeling of pain. Of course, you expect grazes and broken bones to hurt in the short term and, depending on the seriousness of the injury, this will be more or less distressing. You also expect them to get better over time. Some pain and discomfort, however, does *not* seem to get better over time and this can be described as chronic pain.

Chronic pain, such as can occasionally apply to bladder problems, is under the influence of even more factors than the acute pain we have been looking at so far and is even more complicated. When pain is chronic it inevitably has an impact psychologically. That is, you think, feel and act in a certain way about the pain. The nature of these reactions to chronic pain can influence how you cope and the quality

35

of your life. They can also influence those around you who will, in turn, react. This, too, can, in the end, influence the course of the problem. The leap I have just made from a physical pain to a feeling that is influenced by those around you may seem rather unlikely, but I assure you that this is a common scenario. Here is a typical example of what I mean.

David had been having bladder trouble for some time. He had sensations of urgency, but difficulty passing water. It was eventually decided that he needed prostate surgery.

David was at a low ebb. His work was physically demanding and stressful and not well paid – it wasn't even very secure. This had also led to some strains in his relationship with his wife and children.

After the surgery, he was naturally in pain. This made him feel even more down and the thought of going back to work filled him with dread. His wife and children were very supportive and caring. She made sure he took his painkillers, looked after all his needs and cooked his favourite dishes. The children made him cards and presents. If the pain was bad, he would ask for painkillers and take to his bed. His wife was particularly attentive and caring at these times. He still felt tense about going back to work, but, after a couple of weeks, felt he would have to go back.

While at work on that first day, he did not feel particularly well and experienced an excruciating cramping pain in his lower abdomen. He was sent home. His wife was very concerned and his doctor gave him a sick note for another week.

Over time, it becomes more and more difficult for David to return to work and you can see how a pattern is developing that David and his wife could find it difficult to break out of.

Fortunately, David eventually acknowledged his fears about his health and work to his wife, and later to his boss and doctor. They worked out a way for him to return to work gradually, to receive all the medical reassurance he needed and his wife encouraged his positive efforts at slowly getting back to a more balanced lifestyle.

Chronic pain, then, can be affected by psychological factors and general life circumstances. This is supported by the fact that chronic pain and discomfort can vary in intensity over time. It is important to identify the factors that cause these changes. Some may be already clear to you. For example, many of the people I see can make a definite link between feeling 'stressed' and the discomfort worsening. To get a clear idea of the factors influencing discomfort over time, it is essential to keep a diary. This allows you to pay direct attention to the level of discomfort and the interaction of this with other things, such as level of activity, feelings of stress or whatever. You will recall the description of how to keep a diary given in Chapter 1, where you rated your discomfort on a scale of one to ten, initially every hour, and you can use this now, too, making a note of what is happening at that time or including an additional rating of, for example, stress or anxiety, if it is relevant to you.

The three main psychological factors of importance in chronic pain are:

- depression
- tension
- attention

and so I will now describe each of these in turn.

Depression

It has been found that those who suffer chronic pain and discomfort are often depressed. Naturally there has been a chicken and egg-type debate about which comes first. Overall, the conclusion seems to be that the two interact together. It is important to recognize if you are depressed as this is one factor that brings on pain sensations and will also have an enormous influence on how you are able to tackle your health problems. On top of this, depression is easily tackled itself, given the appropriate support. So, what exactly is depression?

Do you frequently

- feel downhearted and sad
- feel at your worst in the morning
- have crying spells
- have trouble getting off to sleep
- wake up too early
- have no appetite
- notice you are losing weight
- feel tired/irritable

- find it hard to do things
- feel hopeless
- find it difficult to enjoy anything?

If a few of these apply to you and you have felt like this for some time, it is important that you visit your doctor to talk about how you have been feeling. The sooner you tackle depression the better because, over time, it is possible to feel more and more hopeless and helpless as a result of the downward spiral that develops – you feel tired and low and therefore do less and therefore feel more negative and so on. Your doctor may suggest you talk to a counsellor or psychologist or may prescribe some antidepressant medication.

Depression is a very common problem, particularly in those with chronic health problems (around 30–40 per cent of people) and an understandable reaction to such difficulties. So you are not alone and the problem can be solved. Try to think about whether the depression is mostly to do with your bladder problems and came on after these difficulties arose or whether you were already depressed before.

If you feel your life is limited by your symptoms:

- take a positive approach to overcoming them
- remind yourself of your achievements and the things you can do
- ask yourself if you are really limited by your symptoms or by your own fears
- remember that having bladder problems in no way affects your worth as a person unless you let it
- don't dwell on things you can't do or how things have changed but make positive plans and take a step at a time.

There are other factors in people's lives that can add to feelings of depression or a lack of self-worth. For example, problems in a significant relationship or stress at work. It could be that on-going tension of this kind is compounding your symptoms and feelings of depression. (I consider stress further in Chapter 9.)

Some people have experienced very traumatic events, either in childhood or their adult lives, such as bereavement, a serious accident or illness, or mistreatment, in whatever way, at the hands of others. Often they have not had the opportunity to come to terms with what has happened and they can end up feeling stressed and depressed later in life. If you think that this applies to you, it is important that you try to find some appropriate help. Doctors are aware of the counselling services available to you locally.

Sometimes it is difficult to accept that physical distress is linked to emotional factors, particularly if the memories are very painful. As a psychologist working with people who have chronic health problems this is something that I encounter every day and I am often struck that people have never told those close to them about experiences that have had a huge impact on their lives and on their feelings. To come to terms with some experiences, it is essential to work with someone else, someone who is experienced and professional and who you trust.

We have seen that it is possible to feel depressed about adjusting to the limitations your symptoms bring or about other aspects of your life. However, the feelings will affect your bladder problems in two ways: making any discomfort feel worse and making it difficult to cope practically and emotionally. Depression is about the meaning you give to your symptoms. If in your heart of hearts you believe that your bladder problems have ruined your life or affect your worth as a person, then you will feel depressed, no matter how hard you try to battle on. Admit to yourself if this is how you really feel and then challenge these ideas by collecting all the evidence against them.

Another meaning that people give to their symptoms is that they are harmful. This naturally leads to feelings of tension and anxiety. Tension is the second factor that can 'turn on' pain and discomfort.

Tension

As with depression, you may be tense or stressed. Again, this can occur because of your symptoms ('I wonder if there is something serious wrong with me', 'What if I can't find a toilet') or because of other aspects of your life ('It will be a catastrophe if I get the sack'). However the tension and stress has arisen, it will make your symptoms and any discomfort worse. Stress is a physical reaction (I discuss it in more detail in Chapter 9, and how to learn to relax in Chapter 10).

If you have worries about your symptoms, then you probably need some reassurance from your doctor. If you have worries about your bladder letting you down, then you could follow the self-help advice given in this book. You may also ask yourself 'What is the worst thing that could happen?' People often react emotionally because they are thinking how terrible something is: 'It would be terrible to be incontinent while I was out shopping'. This leads to you feeling stressed while you are out and worried about the state of your bladder, which will lead to more bladder sensations and more worry and so on (see Figure 5.1).

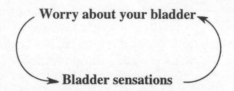

Figure 5.1 The vicious circle of tension and bladder problems

Ask yourself:

● How likely is the thing I fear?
● Has it happened before?
● If it did happen, what would be so terrible?
● What is it that I really fear?

Often what people really fear is not the event itself, but what the event might mean for them. For example, a very sociable person who feels good about themselves when their relationships with others are going well and who likes to be seen as a confident, coping person may really fear that people will reject them because of their problems. Would your friends really abandon you under these circumstances? How would you react if this happened to someone else? Is this situation really terrible or just not very nice? Try to be honest to yourself about what it is that you really fear and then ask yourself how likely this is and would it really be a total catastrophe.

Just as you can get into a downward spiral with depression, so you can get into an upward spiral with tension and discomfort – you feel tense because you are in pain, which makes the pain worse, which makes the tension worse and so on. The more you worry about the symptoms, the worse they will get. This is partly because by worrying about them you are paying attention to them. Attention is the third factor that can 'turn on' pain.

Attention

At any one time, we are only able to pay attention to a tiny amount of the information that is available to us for consideration. Also, whatever you are actively attending to will seem, in some ways, 'amplified'. So, for example, if you are sitting watching your favourite TV programme, you are *not* thinking about your Aunt Judy, what the weather is like or how much you like smoked salmon. You are focused on the plot and the sounds and the imagery of the programme and feeling happy, sad or whatever. If Aunt Judy then telephones you to wish you good luck with your daughter's wedding on Saturday, you may start thinking about the weather and how much you like smoked salmon and the TV programme would then become a faint noise in the background.

The same is true of attention and pain. If you are *focusing* on discomfort, it will be all that is in your mind because it is under the spotlight. If you are distracted by something else, the pain will not be receiving your attention and, for the time being, will not appear as bad (techniques for using this distraction effect to your advantage are described in Chapter 10).

Summary

If you are suffering pain and discomfort and you have the assurance of your doctor that all medical angles have been explored, then you are faced with the prospect of learning to cope with the problems. First, as always, know your enemy. Keep a diary so that you can see what makes it better and worse, then use this knowledge. Is your discomfort influenced by your emotional state, are you depressed or stressed? What do you need to do to reduce these feelings? Do you focus your attention on the discomfort more than is necessary? Use distraction techniques to change this.

6
You are what you drink!

You have lots of information and now we shall put some strategies for tackling the problem into practice.

We touched earlier on the importance of drinking enough liquid of the right sort, and below you will find out now to make necessary changes in your drinking habits if this is applies to you. Changing habits, especially if they are ones that are ingrained, should be a slow process. Something that I cannot emphasize enough is that changes that are made in a steady, progressive way, over a period of time, are more likely to be made permanently than those that you try to make overnight. It is a bit like the hare and the tortoise. It is enough that you are moving in the right direction – do not worry if progress is slow or even if you seem to take a few steps backwards occasionally.

Why drink more liquid?

There are two main reasons for this. The first concerns your general health. There is more water in our bodies than any other substance. All the major bodily functions work best if the body is well hydrated, that is to say when there is enough water. Dehydration can lead to headaches, constipation and other health problems.

The second reason for drinking plenty is more specific and concerns your bladder. The bladder also works best when you are drinking the right amount of fluid. If you drink too little, then the bladder gets used to holding smaller and smaller amounts and becomes more sensitive. Concentrated urine can also irritate the bladder and the urethra. On the other hand, of course, if you drink too much, you will have to visit the toilet more often.

There are a number of reasons people don't drink enough. The first is to do with habit. That is, they have always drunk small amounts, perhaps because they have never been told why they should drink plenty. Alternatively perhaps it is because they lead busy lifestyles and don't always make the time to drink regularly during the day.

The second important reason people don't drink enough is more specific. If you have an irritable bladder and have problems with urgency and frequency, then it seems to make perfect sense to reduce these symptoms by drinking less. In the long term, however, as we have seen, this will only serve to make the bladder more sensitive.

How much should I drink?

The recommended amount is around 1.75 litres (3 pints) of liquid a day. It should be fairly easy for you to work out how much you usually drink. Count up the typical number of mugs and glasses of whatever you would drink in an average day and then measure how much this is by using water and a measuring jug. This will tell you whether or not you are drinking too much or too little in a day. Obviously, the 1.75-litre (3-pint) rule is not a hard and fast one. It depends to a certain extent on your size and levels of activity. In very hot countries, for example, it can be necessary to more than double this intake!

When should I drink it?

The answer is regularly throughout the day, but it helps to get into a routine. Try to arrange it so that you are drinking a set amount about every two hours. Of course, it makes sense to drink less in the evenings, for a couple of hours before bedtime, to avoid a disturbed night.

What should I drink?

If you have irritable bladder problems, then it is important that you try to cut out caffeine. Caffeine is a stimulant and will increase the need to urinate. It is also a diuretic, which means that it encourages the kidneys to produce more urine.

Caffeine is found in coffee, tea and some soft drinks, such as colas. If the idea of giving them up fills you with total horror, then decaffeinated versions of all these are available. Also, you can try phasing these alternatives in over time by, for example, alternating them with 'the real thing' or making a coffee that is half and half. Over time, move over to having only the decaffeinated drinks.

Occasionally, people are slightly addicted to caffeine, particularly if they drink more than eight cups of coffee a day. These people will notice 'withdrawal symptoms', such as headaches, if they try to cut down their intake of them too quickly.

The other thing to avoid (at least in excess) is alcohol. This, too, affects the bladder and is a diuretic. In fact, the dehydrating effect of alcohol is one of the main causes of the dreaded hangover.

Cranberry juice is thought to have beneficial effects on the bladder, but, otherwise, the best thing to drink is water. Most of us are not used to drinking water on its own, mineral or otherwise, but it is possible to develop a taste for it. If the idea really appals you then dilute squash or watered-down fruit juice is a good alternative. Try to avoid too much neat fruit juice, though, as it's rather acidic and concentrated. There is a whole range of herbal teas readily available, too, and these can be very refreshing.

Increasing your fluid intake

As mentioned at the start of this chapter, the important thing is to go slowly. If you are worried about urgency and frequency, then increasing your fluid intake too dramatically will demoralize you. The best way to increase your fluid intake is by drinking more. So, if you think that you need to increase overall consumption by 600 ml (1 pint) a day, then that is about three mugfuls. Then, make it your goal to achieve this intake in a month's time. The first week of this month, you could have one extra drink in the middle of the day, each day. The second week you could increase this to include an extra drink in the morning, and so on until you had reached your goal.

To motivate yourself, you could:

- make a clear plan and write it down
- tell someone you are going to make this change
- keep a diary and tick off your progress, reviewing it each week
- promise yourself something if you stick to your plan
- make a note of any benefits you notice.

Be aware that increasing your fluid intake over time may, in the short term, make the urgency and frequency seem worse, although most people find to their surprise that this doesn't happen. If you are particularly worried about increasing your fluid intake, then make sure you begin when you can have a few days at home to see how you get on. Remember, though, that focusing on the problem can make it worse, so it is important to keep yourself occupied.

In the long term, your bladder will learn to cope with holding more, particularly if you combine this with the advice in the next chapter.

We are really looking for benefits over weeks and months rather than days – it is important to change habits slowly.

Decreasing your fluid intake

Sometimes people are drinking too *much* out of habit. For example, it's easy to get into the habit of constantly putting the kettle on for a cup of tea. Occasionally, therefore, problems of urgency and frequency are caused quite simply by drinking too much.

If this is the case for you, keep a record of your intake and make a plan to monitor the number of drinks you have each day as described in the previous section, but, instead of making it your goal to *increase* your intake over the next month, make it your goal to *decrease* it by the necessary amount.

Summary

Sometimes, the fact that you are not drinking enough fluids can have long-term effects on your bladder. It is important to try to reverse these effects slowly. Certain kinds of drinks, such as coffee, tea and fizzy soft drinks, can have an adverse effect on the bladder. Alcohol should also be avoided in excess as it dehydrates the body.

7

Training your bladder

Bladder training is a very simple and extremely successful way of overcoming the problems of urgency, frequency and incontinence. In fact, it is the most commonly used and useful approach to combating them. Here I will describe how you can set up your own programme. As in the last chapter, it is important to make changes in a slow and steady manner if they are to be lasting. I will also describe how you can prepare for any setbacks. At the end of this chapter, I will describe pelvic floor exercises that can be either combined with bladder training or practised separately.

What is bladder training?

Bladder training is quite simply encouraging your bladder to hold more urine for longer. You can train your bladder to do this by steadily increasing the time between visits to the toilet. Quite simple in theory, but not so simple in practice, I can imagine you saying to yourself! Of course to achieve this goal, what you need to be able to do is to resist the urge that you will inevitably get to empty the bladder sooner than you really need to. This is the essence of the problem and the solution. If you can overcome the 'false' messages from your bladder in the short term, eventually it will give up sending them. Your bladder will become less 'irritable' over time. You will be in control of your bladder, your bladder will not control you.

Training your bladder involves the same principles as any other kind of training. Let's take the example of training a new puppy. We all know that if we want to encourage a dog to repeat a certain behaviour, then we reinforce it. So, if it sits when we tell it, we give it a biscuit. Next time, the dog is more likely to sit when we tell it because doing this has been linked with a pleasant thing before. It is also possible to encourage 'bad' behaviour in a dog by reinforcing it without meaning to. Imagine that the dog barked when it was put out in the garden on its own. To stop the dog barking, you let it in. This is a positive state of affairs for the dog, so next time it is put there it is more than likely to start barking again. If it is again let in, then you are 'teaching' the dog that barking will mean its being let in. You have unintentionally reinforced its barking behaviour. If you are determined that your dog should get used to being outside you will have to brace yourself, and your neighbours, to ignore the barking and only let it in after a set time or when it stops barking, so that the 'link' is unlearned.

Back to the bladder, and the same principles apply. If your bladder starts sending strong messages to be emptied (urgency, or the equivalent of the dog barking) and you respond immediately by going to the toilet (letting the dog in), you are encouraging your bladder to send even stronger urges under the same circumstances in the future. The positive state of affairs here is that you get *temporary* relief from the urgency and the worry associated with it. I stress the word temporary because, in the long run, you are encouraging the bladder to be more irritable, just as the dog was encouraged to bark more. So, to stop your bladder 'barking' at you, you need to brace yourself to tolerate the urges and only empty your bladder after a set time or when the urge has subsided. There are various things you can do to help yourself tolerate the urge, which I will discuss in more detail in Chapters 9 and 10, but that is the principle, and it works.

How can I train my bladder?

The very first step is to keep a diary of frequency, if you have not already done so. That is, noting how often you are visiting the toilet during the day and, most importantly, over the period of a few days, what is the *longest* interval between visits to the toilet that you have achieved? This is your starting point.

There won't be a typical figure, but what you do know is that your bladder can certainly go for whatever time the longest interval was without being emptied. Then what you will be doing is setting an interval that you *know* you can achieve and *only* emptying the bladder at those times, ignoring urges to do so in between.

The best place to start is something slightly short of your 'personal best', so that you know you can achieve it. So, if your diary shows that the longest you can hold on is an hour and 45 minutes, then you should choose to start at a set time of an hour and 30 minutes. Don't worry if you think your starting time should be an hour or even 45 minutes – you need a goal that is a bit of a challenge, but not *too* daunting.

The very first day of your programme will involve you only emptying the bladder when the set time is up, not earlier. Also, if you can hold on even longer, you should do so. It is a good idea not to rush to the toilet the minute the time is up, but to resist the first urge. Remember that you are trying to take control of these unwanted urges, so you need to act as if they don't exist if you want them to go away.

You can increase your set time by a few minutes each day if you want. However, this can be a bit confusing and I suggest that you stick to each time for two or three days, or even more, until you are confident about that gap. Then, increase the set time by 15 minutes and, again, do not go to the toilet until the time is up, then resisit the first urge after that and do not rush to the toilet. Then, increase the gap by another 15 minutes once you are happy with that interval and so on.

The programme can be as long or short as you like. What you are aiming for is to be comfortable without emptying your bladder for three hours or more if you can. Some programmes suggest going up to four hours, but I'm not sure many people *without* bladder problems do that, so don't struggle for this goal. It is possible to increase the set time to three hours or more in just two weeks, but there is no *need* to go this fast – in fact, slow changes may be more easy to keep to in the long term.

So, these are the basic principles – you decide when to empty your bladder and you stick to it, despite messages to do so earlier. You increase the amount of time between visits to the toilet as you go along. Every time you ignore an unwanted urge, you are winning the battle.

At night, empty your bladder before going to bed, then try to resist the urge to empty it within the next hour or so before you go to sleep. If you are in the habit of making 'one last visit', even when you've just been, then try relaxation techniques to get to sleep without doing this. If you wake up in the night and need to urinate, it is best just to get up and do so then get back to sleep. This ensures as little disturbance as possible. The efforts you make to control your bladder during the day will eventually pay off in terms of night-time urgency anyway without you having to make a special effort to tackle it.

Hints for success

Support

When you are trying to make changes in your life, it is always much easier to achieve them if you feel supported. It helps if one or two trusted people know what you are trying to do so that they can support and encourage you. I hope you have managed to think of and approach someone who can help.

It is also extremely important to support yourself by:

- focusing on your successes, not your failures
- being patient and realistic about making changes
- not blaming yourself for your difficulties
- rewarding yourself.

Planning

The clearer your plans, the more likely you are to carry them out and achieve your goals. I have not given specific advice on things such as how often to empty the bladder because everyone will need to start from a point that is appropriate to their own circumstances. This does not mean, though, that you should not be specific to yourself because, in fact, this is very important.

Planning and preparation often make all the difference to the success of a venture. Only begin when you are ready Keep your diary first to assess where you need to begin. Buy a special diary or notebook just for the purposes of your programme and write on the first page some things you would like to achieve, like going to the cinema or starting a course. Write down this week's 'personal best' and the set time you have decided on for the first few days of your programme. Continue to keep the diary daily throughout and to write down your best time each week. Keep your supporter informed of progress or any difficulties.

To give the programme the best chance of success, you may want to focus a lot of effort on it in the first week or two. This may mean taking a few days off work or at least organizing things so that there is nothing to prevent you sticking to the programme. Of course, for it to work in the long term, you will need to incorporate the principles of bladder training into your everyday life.

Plan some small goals into your programme as well as the long-term goal. So, for example, if your overall goal is to achieve an interval of three and a half hours, then plan a special prize for when you achieve a two-hours gap, a two and a half-hours gap and so on. These can be whatever you like, so long as you really like it! For example, a special treat for you might be to buy yourself something or watch a favourite video. I am sure you can think of things that will motivate you, but if you do find it difficult to come up with ideas, it may be that you have got out of the habit of treating yourself. This is actually a very important source of motivation, though, so make a list of activities that you have enjoyed in the past or have ever wanted to try and doing this should get the ideas flowing.

Do not begin on the programme until you have planned carefully what it will involve in practical and emotional terms. It may be that you need to consider two more things before you begin. First, if you are worried about resisting the urge to urinate when it arises, then it will help to practise relaxation and distraction techniques before you begin (see Chapter 10). Also, tensing up the pelvic floor muscles can reduce the urge to urinate, so try the exercises at the end of this chapter. Remember, too, that the more attention you focus on the bladder, the more sensations you are likely to notice. Therefore, plan to keep busy and occupied, particularly if you are usually at work and decide to begin the programme at home.

Second, you need to consider whether or not you have come to avoid a number of activities because of your bladder problems. It is often the case that people can keep to the programme at home, but have difficulties at specific times. This may be linked to worry. For example, going out to the shops or travelling may be worrying because of the greater uncertainty about toilets. This leads to worries about the bladder, which lead to more sensations, which may lead to you making frequent visits to the toilet before leaving home. You will need to be particularly careful at these times and may need to anticipate these problems so that you can avoid them. Perhaps you may even need to decide to tackle some such situations directly. When you have had some success with the training programme, you could set yourself a specific target, such as going to a certain shopping centre and, at the same time, sticking to the programme.

Setbacks

Setbacks are *not* setbacks, they are learning experiences! There is always a reason for a setback and it will teach you something about how to make more progress. Therefore, do not be afraid of setbacks.

Here are some common reasons for them occurring.

- *You have difficulty sticking to the programme* right from the start. You may have set your sights too high. Remember, slow and steady, and set yourself achievable targets. Or perhaps you really cannot fit the programme into your lifestyle. In this case, be flexible. Remember that the principles are to resist unwanted urges to urinate and to increase the time between visits to the toilet and these can be worked into any lifestyle. Try to wait for five extra minutes before emptying the bladder or do one more small job before you go. Keep a record of the time between trips and try to improve on your 'personal best' each week. If you apply these ideas, over time, your symptoms will improve.

- *Something unexpected happens* something out of your control. For example, you lose your job or someone in the family becomes ill. At such times you do not have the resources to keep to the programme and, if the stress is great, the problem may be as bad as ever. Cope as best you can and return to the programme when things are more predictable.

- *You make good progress at home, but the symptoms return whenever you go away from home* You need to do two things. First, acknowledge your fears about leaving the safety of home. If they are mostly to do with trusting your bladder while you are out, then you need to plan an additional programme, increasing the time and distance away from home. Practising relaxation and challenging your fears will also help. By challenging your fears I mean talking to yourself in a calming way. So, if you have the anxiety-provoking thought that it would be terrible to get the urge to urinate while out and not be able to find a toilet, ask yourself how likely this really is, remind yourself of your bladder's ability to hold on for however long you have achieved and so on.

- *You make some initial progress, but cannot keep to the programme* Occasionally, bladder problems are linked to anxiety, but the anxiety was not originally to do with the bladder. When this is the case, as you begin to deal with the bladder problem, another problem may emerge. If this is a difficult problem, it can lead to symptoms returning. Perhaps I should give an example.

Jane had always been very shy and relied very much on her mother for support and encouragement. At the age of 18, she began at college. She found that she had to keep rushing to the loo. She began to worry about this and tried to cope by drinking less and emptying her bladder whenever she had the opportunity. She remembered an incident at primary school when she had a slight 'accident' and worried that this would happen again.

Eventually, she gave up college and sought help for her bladder problems. Jane quickly took to the principles of bladder training. However, she had to deal with the setback caused by the realisation that the anxiety that had originally led to the bladder problem was about becoming independent and coping in novel social situations. She began to tackle this by joining an evening class and taking trips out alone during the day to increase her self-confidence.

• *You have great initial success, but slowly slip back into your old ways* Keep another diary and analyse what you are doing. Often people get in the habit of going to the toilet 'just in case' when this really is not necessary. For example, emptying the bladder before leaving home, regardless of how recently they have been or where they are going. It is rare for shops, restaurants or other people's houses to be toilet-free zones. So, always ask yourself whether this trip is really necessary. Do you really have a full bladder or is this merely a habit? Start yourself on a new programme if this seems appropriate.

Pelvic floor exercises

If you have been told or you suspect that pelvic floor muscle weakness plays a part in your bladder problems, doing appropriate exercises may help. In fact, pelvic floor exercises are completely harmless and may be of benefit even with urgency problems. There are two reasons for this. First, there is some evidence that tensing the pelvic floor muscles can help to reduce the sensation of the urge that can be a problem in irritable bladder. Second, there is also evidence that some bladder problems are linked to difficulties relaxing the pelvic floor muscles when urinating. So, learning to tense and relax these muscles at the right time may help you cope with your bladder problems. Following these exercises can also generally increase the circulation around the pelvic area and so may help with bowel problems, such as constipation.

What are the pelvic floor muscles and what do they do?

The pelvic floor muscles act like a taut hammock holding the bladder and bowel in place. Firm pelvic floor muscles prevent incontinence. When you go to the toilet, they relax and, afterwards, they tighten up again. Weak muscles, though, mean that you may leak urine when you exercise, cough, sneeze or laugh.

What causes this weakness? The muscles can sag as a result of childbirth, lack of exercise, persistent coughing or constipation, being overweight, prostate or other surgery or just getting older. In all these cases, and for both men and women, pelvic floor exercises can strengthen the muscles so that they give the correct support again.

How do I exercise my pelvic floor muscles?

Pelvic floor exercises can be very effective if they are practised correctly and persistently. Probably the hardest part is motivating yourself and remembering to do them often enough and over a long enough period of time. It is likely that you will have to practise them for several weeks to notice a big improvement. Somehow you will have to make these exercises part of your everyday routine if you want to get results. The exercises themselves are simple, try the following.

- Sit comfortably, leaning slightly forwards, with your knees a bit apart. Imagine you are actually trying to stop yourself from passing wind. You should feel the pelvic floor muscles tighten and lift, without moving your legs, buttocks or stomach muscles.
- This time, imagine you are stopping the stream of urine mid flow and, again, you should feel the muscles lift.
- Do both these lifts together. You should feel the whole area tighten and lift and this is the effect you want.
- Practise tensing the pelvic floor muscles by tensing and pulling up the muscles slowly and holding them as tight as you can for five seconds, or as long as you can at first, then relaxing them to a count of five. Repeat this process five times. Then, pull up and tense the muscles quickly and relax them immediately in five quick squeezes. That's it, five slow and five quick tenses. Repeat this exercise ten times a day.

You can actually try to stop your flow of urine next time you go to the toilet, half way through emptying your bladder and then relaxing again. You may not be successful if the muscles are weak, but if you are then you know you are tensing the correct muscles when you do the exercises. This test should not be repeated too often as it is important to always ensure that the bladder empties completely. Perhaps try it once a week to assess progress.

Some additional tips

Use tricks to remind yourself to do the exercises, such as doing them every hour, ticking off each time you do them and so on.

It helps to tense up the pelvic floor muscles before you sneeze or cough or if you are trying to resist the urge to urinate.

Some alternatives

If you have difficulties doing the exercises in the correct way or are not having any success, there are a number of other approaches.

- *Cone therapy* This is a fairly new approach for women that has had some good results. You exercise the pelvic floor twice a day for 15 minutes by inserting a cone-shaped weight into the vagina and use the pelvic floor muscles to keep it in place. As the strength of these muscles increases, you can increase the weight of the cone you use. A sort of pelvic floor weight training! The advantage is that you don't have to keep remembering to repeat tensing exercises throughout the day. Cones are becoming more widely available from pharmacies, but if you cannot find any, they can be ordered from the address given in the Useful addresses section at the back of the book.

- *Electrotherapy* This is a way of making the muscle contract using specialist equipment. Electrodes need to be carefully positioned so that an electric current causes the correct stimulation. This kind of treatment is usually carried out by physiotherapists and requires attendance at a clinic. It also requires you to continue practising tensing and relaxing the muscle at home. Its usefulness mostly lies in learning which muscles to contract.

- *Perineometer* This is a piece of equipment that simply gives women feedback about pressure in the vagina so that you can see whether the exercises are being performed correctly. Over time, it can also give you a measure of improvement, which can be very encouraging. Again, this equipment is only available in clinics and success still relies on the long-term correct exercising of the pelvic floor.

Summary

Bladder training involves teaching the bladder to tolerate larger amounts of urine for longer. To do this you need to learn to ignore the urge to empty the bladder and to only do so after a set time. This set time should be increased gradually until you can last up to three to four hours. The programme is flexible and you should design one that's best for you. You may need to learn ways of resisting the urge to empty the bladder, such as relaxation and distraction techniques. Sometimes worries about the bladder or other life problems may need to be tackled before lasting progress can be made.

Strengthening and becoming aware of the pelvic floor muscles can help with bladder symptoms. To really benefit from pelvic floor exercises, you need to practise them every day for several weeks. Cone therapy can offer women an alternative approach to tensing exercises.

8

Health and relationships

In Chapter 4, I discussed a number of factors that can affect how the bladder works. I touched on the fact that the bladder can be influenced by your lifestyle, for example, your diet and how much exercise you get. Such factors are often hard work to change, but you may have little chance of overcoming your bladder difficulties in the long term unless these underlying problems are addressed where necessary. Just as the bladder is influenced by outside factors, so these factors can be influenced by bladder problems. For example, having bladder problems may lead to a restricted lifestyle, which may lead to a lack of exercise, which may lead to weight problems, which may affect the bladder and so on. Just as you have designed a programme of bladder training for yourself, you may need to tackle some of these other problems, too.

The other important area where bladder problems can have an influence is in relationships. Relationships in general can be altered, but sexual relationships may be particularly affected. So, this chapter is about health and relationships.

Diet

We hear a lot about what we should and should not eat. Sometimes it seems like *all* foods are bad for us! We are also bombarded with images of 'perfect' bodies and stories of those whose lives were transformed by losing weight.

All of this information can sometimes lead us to forget about our *own* body's needs. We are all different and there is no ideal diet or weight. This will vary according to your age, lifestyle and build. It is now widely accepted that very low-calorie diets are bad for you in the long run because your body slows down to conserve energy and when you start to eat normal foods you will put on weight again.

The bladder may be adversely affected by being very overweight or by chronic constipation. If these are long-standing problems for you, then it may help to seek some advice and support from your doctor in the first instance. The doctor may refer you to a dietician. Everyone can benefit from an improved diet. Dietary changes can have quite a noticeable effect on mood and energy levels, for example. Here are some important things to remember.

- Habits that you change slowly are more likely to be lasting changes for the better. Crash diets are not the answer because you cannot keep to them for ever – you must be able to live the rest of your life with your eating habits.
- Be flexible. Allow yourself some indulgences. Listen to your body and give it what it needs. Eat small amounts regularly in the day rather than eating a lot at night when you don't need the energy. Make time to plan, prepare and eat meals rather than eating on the run.
- Many of us, particularly women, have problems distinguishing between hunger and emotional states, such as upset and anger. This is often learned at a very early age and can lead to problems of over- or undereating. Recognize if this applies to you and try to learn new ways of dealing with emotional situations.
- The best general advice is to make sure you have enough fibre in your diet to prevent constipation (fruit, vegetables and high-fibre cereals) and cut down on fats (cheese, cream, butter) and refined sugars (sweets, chocolate, cake) wherever possible. When you go shopping, take a list and don't buy high-fat and high-sugar content products. If they are not in the house, you are less likely to eat them!
- Occasionally, cases of irritable bladder have been helped by a gluten-free diet. If you suspect that you have a food allergy, ask your doctor for advice and help.
- Foods that increase the acidity of your urine can irritate the bladder and may encourage infection, particularly in women. To avoid this, do not drink excessive quantities of alcohol, cut out caffeine, don't eat too much citrus fruit or soft fruits like strawberries, and don't eat large amounts of spicy foods. You can reduce the acidity of urine by drinking plenty of water.

Exercise

Many of us fail to exercise enough. This can be because of busy lifestyles, which leave us too exhausted mentally and too short of time to contemplate exercise, or because of a restricted lifestyle, where exercise is avoided because of bladder worries.

Taking adequate amounts of exercise is important for general health, mood and specific problems, such as weakened muscles. Exercise does not have to be torture to be beneficial. Do not let memories of PE lessons at school put you off.

As with dietary changes, the main mistake that people make is to try to do too much too soon, only ending up discouraged. You are not aiming for the Olympics! The important thing is to make small, but lasting changes.

Gentle exercise can be very relaxing and have positive effects on your feelings of well-being. There is no lifestyle that excludes all forms of exercise. You do not need to spend a fortune on expensive equipment and gym fees and miss your lunch hours trying to fit in a game of squash. Walking is one of the best forms of exercise. Simply walking for ten minutes, three times a week and building up week by week until you reach half an hour, three times a week, will make a big difference. Make sure you allow yourself the time and perhaps enlist a companion or take a little cassette player along if that encourages you.

If you have particular health problems that make it difficult to exercise in this way, then it might be worth asking to see a physiotherapist for some individual advice. If you are worried about exercising because of bladder problems, then remember that the long-term effect of exercising in terms of mood and muscle tone will be beneficial and that you do not have to do particularly strenuous movements to keep fit. In fact, the walking programme may kill two birds with one stone – increasing your fitness and overcoming fears of being away from home for increasing periods of time.

Hygiene and clothing

There are some simple, effective tips women can follow to avoid bladder infection and genital irritation.

- Shower regularly rather than bath. Use gentle soaps not highly scented ones as these can irritate this sensitive area. Don't use deodorants or disinfectants in this area for the same reason.
- Avoid tight clothing. Tight jeans and other clothes will put unwanted pressure on the bladder. Wear cotton underwear and avoid nylon tights, especially in summer, as the dampness they create can encourage fungal infections.
- Always take the time to empty your bladder and bowels completely and without rushing.

- It is a good idea to empty the bladder both before and after sex. This ensures that if you have problems of urgency or leakage, you are more able to relax with your partner as your bladder is empty. For those with a history of cystitis, one of the main causes of bladder infection is bacteria being encouraged up the urethra during intercourse, but these are flushed out by emptying the bladder afterwards, minimizing the chances of an infection occurring. If you are particularly prone to infections, then showering or rinsing the genital area before and after sex as well is also advisable. This may all sound like a lot of effort, but those who have suffered the misery of bladder infections will know that *any* means of avoiding it is worth its weight in gold!

Intimate relationships

Irritable bladder problems can affect your sexual relationships in a number of ways. We all know that worries and distractions of any kind can interfere with the relaxation and enjoyment that you can achieve with your partner. This can lead to tension in a relationship that, if not resolved, can, over time, lead to further problems, such as an avoidance of intimate situations. Worries that can interfere with intimacy are usually related to the bladder problem in some way. For example, you might worry that your partner thinks less of you because of the bladder problems or about the bladder symptoms themselves, such as urgency.

In the first instance, it can obviously be terribly difficult to bring up these worries with your partner. However, sometimes voicing your fears is all that is needed to clear the air and allow you to relax again. Also, actively put relaxation techniques into practice and try to focus your attention on sensations other than those coming from the bladder. Worrying about urgency only makes it worse.

If it has been difficult to talk over your worries about sexual situations for a long period of time, you may have got to the stage of almost complete avoidance. In this case, an open discussion and agreement about gradually experimenting with greater intimacy is probably the best way forward.

Empty your bladder before sex. If you are worried about incontinence, try putting a towel over the sheet and remember that urine is sterile and odourless when it leaves the body.

Occasionally, people have specific sexual difficulties, either related to the bladder problem or that were there before, for example, impotence or premature ejaculation in men and vaginismus or difficulty reaching orgasm in women. All these difficulties are also made worse by worry and anxiety, but they can all be overcome given the appropriate advice. Unfortunately it is beyond the scope of this book to give such advice here, but there are many good books available if you think that this applies to you or your partner.

As with other aspects of bladder problems covered earlier, bladder and sexual worries can be made worse by worry and this worry is often about the problem itself, so that vicious circle gets going. Tackling the problem *and* the worry together, therefore, is the best strategy. Sometimes, on the other hand, the worry that is adding to the problem is related to something else. So, for example, if you are very stressed at work, you may have trouble relaxing in a sexual situation, you may then worry about this, which will add to your difficulty relaxing in future sexual situations. Sometimes, the original stress situation also needs to be resolved. Is it possible that stress in one area of your life is affecting both your bladder and your relationships? What needs to be tackled?

It is not uncommon for relationship difficulties themselves to be a major source of stress that can influence bladder and sexual problems. If your relationship is already strained, it will be difficult to overcome these. What needs to be tackled?

Sexual violence is very difficult to talk about and can remain a hidden trauma for many women and also men. Yet, it has been a reality for large numbers of people at some stage in their lives. Obviously, such experiences have wide-ranging influences on relationships and sexuality. If such experiences were a reality for you and you feel your relationships are affected by them, I would encourage you to find the appropriate help you need to recognize how to break this influence. This may be a very hard step to take, but the only one that will take you forward.

Summary

Your bladder is influenced by your general health and emotional well-being. Sometimes there are steps you have to take to improve these before your bladder problems can be overcome.

Slow and steady changes in diet and exercise will be easier to keep to and will bring long-term benefits.

Bladder worries can have an adverse effect on close relationships. Discussing these problems is often avoided because of embarrassment, but tackling the difficulty is the only lasting solution.

9

Stress and the bladder

As we now know, the bladder is clearly influenced by stress, 'nerves' and worry. This is true for everyone, but can be a particular problem for some people. Stress leads to a feeling of urgency that can trick you into thinking that you need to empty your bladder when you don't really. Think of times you've visited the toilet before an important event only to find that you didn't really need to go after all. Being nervous has stimulated the bladder, we have worried about needing the toilet, so have rushed there to try to relieve the feeling. When the 'nerves' have passed and the 'big event' is over, then, usually, you are no longer aware of the urgency feeling. Of course, if you are stressed a lot of the time or it is the bladder problem itself that is stressful for you, then this sense of urgency can become a longer-term problem.

So, what do we mean by 'stress', what are the signs of stress, how can you tell if it is playing a part in your irritable bladder problems and, most importantly, what can be done to reduce it?

What is stress?

Stress is one of those modern words that we hear so often we think we know what it means. The fact is that there are many different ways of understanding and defining stress. Even psychologists who specialize in this area continue to disagree about how best to define it!

There are three main ways of thinking about stress. The first is that things in the world are stressful and stress us. So stress is 'out there'. This is what people mean when they talk about 'stressful life events'. What kinds of events are stressful? They are events that involve a change of some kind, such as moving house, changing job or having a baby. As you can see from these examples, the events do not have to be bad things to be stressful. Generally, the more changes you have to cope with at any one time and the less control you have over the changes, the more stressed you are likely to be. Other factors that can add to stress levels can be on-going problems, such as money worries or relationship difficulties. These are often called 'strains'. One thing that can protect people against the stress of coping with the changes that come with such 'life events' and on-going strains is social support. Social support means having good-quality relationships with family, friends or colleagues that allow you to talk through problems, get information and decide how to handle things for the best.

Although these ideas are very useful, there is one problem with this way of looking at stress. It is that the same stressful life events and strains never have exactly the same effect on two different people. So, Theresa may find public speaking extremely stressful whereas Gillian may actively enjoy it. So seeing *events* as stressful is not a perfect explanation of stress.

The second way of looking at stress is to think about the signs of stress in a person. The effects of stress can be broken down into short-term and long-term effects. When a person is in some immediate danger, the alarm reaction – or 'fight or flight' response – is automatically triggered. You will know what this response feels like if you have ever had a near miss road accident or some such experience. In the longer term, stress can have more wide-ranging effects on how we feel, behave, think and how our bodies work. These are described in more detail later.

The trouble with this second approach is that we may be able to see what it is like to be stressed, but we don't understand why this happens or know what to do about it. Seeing stress as wholly 'out there' as the life events and strains of the first approach or 'in here' as the effects of stress in the second does not get us very far.

The best, third way to think about stress puts both these ideas together. As human beings, we are constantly trying to solve problems and perform well in the world. We and others make constant demands on us to work well, look after others and so on. Up to a certain point, these demands are helpful to us and achieving our goals makes us feel more confident. However, when we think that the demands (life events and strains) placed on us are too great for us to cope with, then we experience stress. So, the way we cope in the face of such demands and how many demands we put on ourselves will determine how stressed we are. The important point here, therefore, is that stress is a very individual thing. There are no universal rules about stress because:

- *We put demands on ourselves* Of course, the world is often unpredictable and stressful life events happen, like losing a job or someone close to us dying, but, for the most part, we put demands on ourselves. For example, I should work late, I should help others more, I must get that promotion. Such demands are very individual. They are a result of what we think of as our role and purpose in life, which, in turn, are a result of a complicated process of socialization.

- *We experience stress when we think that we cannot cope* This means that, in the face of a problem, we might feel that we don't have the ability to manage emotionally or practically. We may feel this way for a number of reasons, because of the way we have handled similar problems in the past or lack of knowledge or lack of support or whatever. If we can solve a problem, sidestep it or accept it, then we do not experience stress.

I expect you are wondering how all this has anything to do with your bladder problem. It is important in two ways. First, if you feel you are not coping with the demands placed on you, then you will experience feelings of stress. As we have seen, one effect of this is for bladder symptoms to worsen. Second, bladder problems themselves place a high demand on your ability to cope. This is made worse by the taboo around the subject. People do not have information about how to understand their problem and how to cope effectively because it is hard to talk about it. Because it is hard to talk about it, people do not feel supported. The problem remains because it is hidden and the stress remains because the problem is not solved.

In a nutshell, we feel unpleasantly stressed when we feel that the demands on us are too great.

Are you stressed?

A certain amount of stress is a good thing – it can be very motivating and invigorating. Indeed, some people seem to almost thrive in high-stress situations. However, stress can also be unpleasant. Here are some of the unpleasant effects of stress.

Physical effects

- *In the short term* Increased heart and breathing rate, dizziness, sweating, blushing, shakes, nausea, butterflies, frequent urination, diarrhoea.
- *In the long term* All the above plus high blood pressure, chest pain, headaches, migraine, stomach ulcers, bladder and bowel problems.

How you think

• Problems of concentration, difficulty making decisions, worrying, being overly self-critical, irrational ideas, fearfulness.

What you do

• You avoid stressful situations, avoid talking to people, drink and smoke too much, eat more (or less), go off sex, get irritable with people, have problems sleeping.

How can stress cause so many different symptoms?

Imagine that someone has just thrown a hand grenade into the room where you are sitting. Knowing immediately that you are in danger, adrenalin is pumped around the body. This is the 'fight or flight' response. Also, breathing increases and the heart beats faster to supply lots of oxygen to the muscles in your legs so that you can run away very fast. Blood is diverted from non-essential areas to the major muscles, this is the explanation for the butterflies sensation as digestion is not your immediate problem! You are ready to spring into action and run away.

We all have this mechanism and it is very important that we do so that we can get out of danger. Of course, most situations that we see as threatening in modern life cannot be solved by fighting or running away. For example, if you are in danger of losing your job and this is a threatening state of affairs for you, your body will react with this stress response, but you cannot solve the problem by literally running or fighting. As long as you see the situation as threatening, your body will react with this stress response. The longer the problem goes on, then the more effects this will have on your health and well-being.

People find different things stressful and also feel the effects of stress differently. Try to think about the situations that you find stressful. Do they have anything in common? Is it possible to say what it is that makes these situations stressful for you? Is there anything you could learn or do to reduce your fears? How do you feel when you are stressed, that is, which particular symptoms do you experience? Can you identify any links between stressful situations and irritable bladder symptoms?

We now know that we experience stress when we see danger or threat of any kind. This does not have to be a physical threat, like someone throwing a hand grenade at you, it could be a threat to your self-esteem or health. This is how bladder problems, particularly incontinence, can be stressful. Such problems are often experienced as a major threat to self-esteem.

How to tackle stress

As we have discussed, unpleasant stress occurs when we think of a situation as threatening. The three ways of tackling stress are thus as follows.

- *Take some direct action that solves the problem* Taking the example of being likely to lose your job, direct action might include trying to find another job. If we take bladder problems as an example of potential threat to self-esteem and health, then direct action might include going to the doctor, following self-help advice and so on. If there are just too many demands on you in general, prioritize, give things up, lower your standards a bit, ask other people to help you, plan some time for yourself. We all need time to unwind if we are to function at our best. Make sure you take proper breaks during the day and relax on days off. The body is a complicated machine that needs regular tending to work well. You should try to have at least an hour to yourself each day to relax and do the things you enjoy. If all of this seems impossible, then you need to think about your lifestyle and what you are trying to achieve. Sometimes choosing not to reduce the demands on yourself means choosing to be stressed. If you find it hard to say 'No' to people, you may often find yourself overloaded. Women in particular often feel uncomfortable about putting themselves first. Unfortunately, the problem with always putting *others* first is that you end up feeling stressed and exhausted. Make it a goal to become more assertive – buy a book on the topic or join a local group. Being able to talk through problems is often an essential part of solving them and keeping them in perspective. Have you lost touch with old friends and work colleagues? How can you go about starting to build some social support for yourself?
- *Think as realistically as possible about the situation* Try to avoid making emotional responses to problems before you have all the information you need to understand the difficulty. Because a situation *feels* hopeless it does not mean that it *is* hopeless. Catastrophizing ('This is a terrible situation') and self-blame ('It's all my fault that this has happened') are very demotivating and stop

you looking for solutions. What really is the worst thing that can happen and is it that bad? What resources do you have or could you create to help you? All problems can also be opportunities for learning, growth and change. What are the good things that could come out of this difficulty? People are more likely to think in very negative terms about situations that all of us fear, such as embarrassment, loss of control or illness. It is not surprising, therefore, that irritable bladder sufferers are worried about their symptoms. All the more reason to be as objective as possible about the situation.

- *Learn ways of keeping calm* Learning to keep calm is a skill that takes a lot of practice to achieve. It involves recognizing signs of stress, learning to relax and noticing and challenging thinking that can make situations seem more stressful ('It would be awful if . . .', 'I would just die if . . .', etc.). Some ways of relaxing and keeping calm are described in the next chapter.

The stress of bladder problems

Naturally, many people are worried about their bladder problems. As we know, stress can affect the bladder, so how can these worries be overcome?

The first thing is to get as much information as you can about the problem (this might be from reading, or talking to healthcare professionals). Find out what can be done to help you and what you can do for yourself. Talk through the problem with someone supportive, follow the advice given in this book. Do not blame yourself for your difficulties – bladder problems are nothing to be ashamed of. Try to tackle difficult situations and changes in lifestyle a step at a time.

Summary

This chapter has outlined the essentials of understanding and managing stress. If you wish to find out more, there are plenty of books devoted to the subject and they can be very helpful. See the Further reading system at the end of the book. If you think you are having considerable problems with anxiety, for example panic attacks, and avoiding many situations, then you should consider talking to your GP who may be able to put you in touch with someone, such as trained nurse, counsellor or psychologist, who can help you to look at your particular problems and gradually overcome them.

10

Learning to relax

The title of this chapter is so named because I wish to emphasize that the techniques described are only helpful if they are practised a lot! Just as it would be impossible for me to wake up tomorrow morning as a concert pianist, so it is impossible to instantly become a totally stress-free and relaxed person. This is especially the case if your levels of stress and tension have been building up over many years. Once you have mastered the basic techniques, though, you can put them into practice in everday life so that, as time goes by, you get better at keeping your stress under control. So, why is it good to relax, how can you learn to relax and what other techniques can be useful?

Why relax?

When you are relaxed, you are in the opposite state, physically and mentally, to that of when you are stressed. The physical sensations are pleasant. You breathe calmly, your heart beats more slowly, your blood pressure falls, your muscles are relaxed. The psychological effects are enjoyable. You feel an inner calm, there are pleasant thoughts and images in your mind, you can think more rationally. Over time, you may sleep better, feel less tired, get fewer headaches and general aches and pains and, hopefully, fewer irritable bladder problems. In fact, a number of small studies on the subject have found that relaxation is very useful in the treatment of bladder problems. I have also seen this for myself in many patients, who can link their symptoms to stress or find themselves tensing up all the time. Discomfort and worrying about a particular part of the body can lead you instinctively to protect it by tensing up the muscles around that area. This is why those suffering from irritable bladder often report aches and pains in the lower back, abdomen and legs. Therefore, learning to release that tension can reduce the discomfort and improve symptoms. Another important reason for being in favour of relaxation is that it has no unwanted side-effects!

How to relax

We all have activities that we find relaxing, such as having a long hot bath or watching TV. What these activities usually have in common is that we are relatively still, there are no demands on us and our minds are occupied with something pleasant. These are the essentials of relaxation and you can learn to provide them for yourself any place, any time – with a bit of practice!

To begin with, read through the rest of this chapter. As before it is not always easy to change habits and if you progress in gradual steps you are more likely to be successful than if you try to achieve your goal too quickly. The more planning and commitment you put into any change the more likely you are to succeed.

You will get the most benefit from practising relaxation if you set aside half an hour each day for regular sessions. I can imagine some of you gasping at this, thinking that it's impossible. If this is the case, then your first task is to work out how you are going to find this time. After lunch, when you get home from work or just before bedtime? Furthermore, you need to ensure that you have a quiet, warm room where you will not be disturbed. Make sure other people in the house know this is your time, take the phone off the hook and hang a 'do not disturb' sign on the door! The other thing you need is a comfortable place to lie with your head slightly supported, this can be on the bed or in a comfortable armchair.

There are a number of kinds of relaxation techniques, but they all have three parts in common. The first is calm breathing, and this should always be how you start a relaxation session. The second is concentrating on muscle tension in the body and releasing it. The third is holding calming images in the mind.

The reason for these stages is that each adds to the relaxation. When we are stressed, we often breathe poorly. Relaxed breathing can lead to an immediate feeling of well-being. Muscle tension is a central effect of being stressed and leads on to many of its other harmful effects, so it is important to learn how to let this go. Last, as we have discussed, stress symptoms in the body are often triggered by how we are thinking about a situation. If your mind is full of stressful thoughts, such as 'I must do so and so or else . . .', 'It is terrible/awful that . . .', 'I'll never manage . . .', then your body will respond with a stress reaction. If your mind is full of pleasant thoughts and images, such as a favourite memory, a beautiful scene or a pleasant fantasy or daydream, then your body responds by relaxing.

70

I am going to describe each of the three stages, breathing, relaxing away tension and thinking calm thoughts. Different people prefer different parts of this process and you may find that you benefit particularly from, say, the breathing practice. Practise each of the parts separately and together and see what works best for you.

Relaxation is becoming much more popular these days as people acknowledge its benefits for health and well-being. It is easy to buy audio tapes of relaxation training. They are widely available from booksellers, healthfood shops and by mail order. Following a tape is often a good way of ensuring that you set aside enough time to relax completely. Not all tapes are the same and you may have to try a couple before you find the right one for you. Self-hypnosis tapes usually combine calm breathing and visualization and some people benefit from this form of relaxation. Although calm breathing and muscle relaxation can be practised almost anywhere, imagery and visualization should only be practised as part of a complete relaxation session, when you are lying or sitting peacefully. Do *not* listen to relaxation tapes, self-hypnosis tapes or practise imagery as you are driving!

A breathing exercise

Sit or lie comfortably and fully supported. Place one or both hands lightly on your stomach, close your eyes and breathe through your nose. Breathe slowly and deeply. Your stomach should rise and fall as you breathe in and out. This breathing should come naturally and not be an effort.

As you breathe in, feel the stomach rising; as you breathe out say the word 'calm' to yourself. As you breathe out, breathe any tension away and allow your body to relax.

You should feel more relaxed, heavier and calmer. Practising this for ten minutes a day can lead to an increased feeling of calm.

Relaxing away muscle tension

Some people find that the breathing exercise is enough to relax their bodies and muscles completely, but if your body is very tense or there are specific areas of muscle tension, then these may need direct attention.

Muscles will relax more if they are tensed up first and then relaxed, and this can be repeated to improve results. Tensing and relaxing also draws your attention to the muscular effects of stress and you may

71

then recognize it happening as you go about your everyday life, so you can then release tension before it builds up.

Some people find it useful to go through the whole body, tensing and relaxing the major muscle groups as part of their relaxation procedure, while others may choose to focus on a selection of specific muscles. The muscle groups most affected by tension are those in the neck and shoulders.

Sit or lie comfortably with your hands by your sides and your legs slightly apart. Close your eyes.

Take a deep breath in and breathe out slowly, saying the word 'calm' to yourself as you do so. Keep breathing slowly and regularly throughout.

For each muscle group given below, inhale, tense those muscles for a count of five, then breathe out and relax them. Focus on the relaxed muscles and then repeat once. The sequence for tensing the muscles is as follows:

- for the hand you write with, make a tight fist
- for the other hand, repeat
- for the upper arm, press your elbow back into the chair or bed
- for the other upper arm, repeat
- for the face, clench your jaw, wrinkle your nose and wrinkle your forehead
- for the neck, press your head back against the chair or into the pillow
- for the shoulders and chest, take a deep breath, push your chest out and your shoulders back
- for the stomach, pull your muscles in
- for the thighs, tense them up, and, if you are sitting, press your heels into the floor
- for the calves and feet, point your toes away and curl them down.

When you have completed this sequence, focus for a few minutes on how the relaxed muscles feel and the sense of calm.

This sequence is easier to follow while listening to a tape as you don't have to think what to do next. If you have any difficulties tensing and relaxing any muscles or any pain, then leave them out of the sequence and concentrate more on the breathing and visualization exercises.

A visualization exercise

When you have learned to feel relaxed using breathing and muscle relaxation, then move on to visualization.

Choose a calm scene, either one from memory or one you can imagine. It could be anything, the most important thing is that you find it relaxing. For example, you might like to visualize yourself on a beach, curled up by a log fire or in the country. You should use all your senses to get absorbed in the scene, thinking about what can you see (colours, people, movement), hear (birds, water, wind, voices), touch (textures, temperatures) and smell (flowers, the sea).

Begin in the same position as the last two exercises, sitting or lying comfortably, closing your eyes and focusing on calm breathing. As you breathe out, say the word 'calm' to yourself.

Begin to imagine the scene you have chosen in your mind's eye. Try to imagine as much detail as you can, as if you were actually there. If your mind drifts off from it, bring yourself back gently to the scene. It can take a lot of practice to keep your mind focused on it. Continue visualizing the scene for ten minutes or so.

Some hints

These three ways of relaxing – the breathing, the muscle relaxation and the visualization – can be practised separately or together. Keep practising until you find what works best for you and then practise your chosen exercise(s) regularly. Allow yourself time to relax completely and get up slowly at the end of a session after taking a couple of really deep breaths.

Put the principles into practice in real life. If you feel yourself tensing up, relax the tension away (particularly when it occurs in the neck and shoulders), by breathing calmly and repeating the word 'calm' to yourself as you breathe out. Ten minutes spent on these techniques in the middle of a hectic day can make all the difference to your stress levels.

Relaxation and irritable bladder

Learning to relax will help you to cope with your bladder symptoms and may directly improve them. Some people may have fears about relaxing and letting go, especially if they have been tense for a long time or they believe that the tension is protecting them in some way.

73

If you have fears of incontinence, it is likely that you instinctively tense up your pelvic floor muscles, buttocks and stomach. Try a gradual programme of tensing and relaxing these muscle groups and remember to relax them if you feel yourself tensing up during the day. If you have weak pelvic floor muscles you should consciously tense up the area before coughing, sneezing, laughing or lifting and then relax them again afterwards. Sometimes squeezing your pelvic floor muscles can help you resist the urge caused by an unwanted bladder contraction.

If you are training your bladder and trying to ignore the urge to pass water, then relaxation can help you with this. Focus on breathing and relaxation as a distraction from the sensations, repeating the word 'calm' to yourself. Practise the visualization exercise, too, and use this for five or ten minutes when you want to delay emptying your bladder. Remember that if you focus on discomfort, then it feels worse. Here are some distraction techniques.

Distraction techniques

- *Focus on the world around you* Look in great detail at things around you.
- *Focus on a particular object* Choose an object that has very happy associations for you, such as a photograph or souvenir. Focus on it and use it as a link into pleasant thoughts and memories.
- *Mind games* Do a crossword, recite poetry, think of a boy's and a girl's name for each letter of the alphabet, listen to a language tape and try to learn new phrases, anything that takes your mind off it.
- *Action* Go for a short walk, do a household job, bake a cake, write a letter. Make a list of activities you enjoy that you can refer to when you need to be distracted.

The principle behind such strategies is that it will be easier for you to resist unwanted urges and so make your bladder calmer in the future if you are not focused on and worried about it. Distracting your attention from your bladder using any of the above ideas or whatever works best for you will enable you to achieve this end.

Summary

Relaxation can be extremely beneficial. To get the maximum benefit, make it part of your daily routine and put it into practice in stressful situations.

LEARNING TO RELAX

Relaxation involves calm breathing, relaxing muscle tension and focusing thoughts on a pleasant scene. These techniques and other ways of distracting your attention can be helpful in bladder retraining as they allow you to more easily resist the urge to empty the bladder.

A few final words

I hope that you have found the advice in this book helpful. Irritable bladder problems are much more common than you would expect and can develop for a number of reasons. The key points made in the book are summarized below. I wish you every success in coping with your irritable bladder.

Be aware of your symptoms
Liquids; drink plenty, avoid caffeine
Attitude; think positive
Delay bladder emptying
Distraction techniques; use them to draw attention away from the bladder
Exercise the pelvic floor muscles
Relax!

Relationships are important supports
Unfulfilled ambitions; fulfil them!
Lifestyle; diet, hygiene and fitness
Expect to fail sometimes, it's ok
Stress management

Glossary of medical terms

Abdomen The belly or tummy.

Anus The opening of the bowel in your bottom, which is controlled by sphincter muscles.

Bladder training A programme to increase the time gap between trips to the toilet to improve bladder capacity.

Cystitis An infection of the bladder.

Cystoscopy A visual examination of the inside of the bladder by means of a very small camera passed up the urethra under general or local anaesthetic.

Detrusor muscle The muscle in the wall of the bladder.

Diuretic A substance that encourages the production of urine.

Hysterectomy The surgical removal of the womb.

Incontinence Involuntary loss of urine.

Menopause Hormonal changes in women, usually between 45 and 55, when periods cease.

Micturition Passing urine to empty the bladder.

Prolapse Descent of the pelvic organs due to a weakening of the supporting muscles.

Prostate It surrounds the urethra just below the bladder neck in men and is a gland that produces fluid for semen.

Sphincter A circular band of muscle that regulates the passage of fluids or solids through a tube.

Unstable bladder A bladder that contracts on filling, causing a sudden and urgent desire to pass urine.

Ureters Thin tubes that run from the kidneys to the bladder.

Urethra The tube leading from the bladder to the outside world, about 5 cm (2 inches) long, in females and running through the penis in males.

Urodynamics Tests to study the behaviour of the bladder on filling and emptying.

Useful addresses

The Continence Foundation
2 Doughty Street
London WC1N 2PH
Tel: 0171–404 6875

Colgate Medical Ltd,
Shirley Avenue
Windsor
Berkshire
SL4 5LH
Tel: 01753 860378

Suppliers of vaginal cones by mail order.

Incontinence Information Helpline
2 pm – 7 pm weekdays
Tel: 0191–213 0050

Further Reading

Cystitis:
Kilmartin, Angela, *Understanding Cystitis: A complete self-help guide to overcoming thrush and cystitis.* Arrow Books 1989.

Stress:
Tyrer, Dr Peter, *How to Cope with Stress.* Sheldon 1980.
Cooper, C. *Living with Stress.* Penguin Health 1988.

Assertion:
Gutmann, Joanna, *The Assertiveness Workbook.* Sheldon 1993.
Smith, Manuel, *When I Say No I Feel Guilty.* Bantam Books 1989.

General:
Burns, David, *Feeling Good: The new mood therapy.* Avons Books 1980.

Sexual relationships:
Hooper, Ann, *Women and Sex.* Sheldon Press 1987.

Index